Sleeping with ED

Victoria Lehmann
and
Michael Kirby

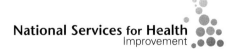

National Services for Health
Improvement

Published in the UK by:
National Services for Health Improvement
Nucleus@The Bridge, London Science and Business Park
Brunel Way, Dartford, Kent DA1 5GA

Copyright 2008 National Services for Health Improvement
Printed in the UK by Nuffield Press Ltd
Funded by Pfizer Limited

ISBN 978-0-9554803-0-0

Any product mentioned in this book should be used in accordance with the prescribing information prepared by the manufacturer. Neither the author nor the publisher can accept responsibility for any detrimental consequences arising from the information contained herein.

A catalogue record for this book is available from the British Library.

Contents

Dedications

Victoria

To my very special Daniel, Samuel and Lucy. I love you all very much and to see you smiling gives me the greatest joy of all.

Mike

To my wife Sue and children Tiffany and Matthew, for always being there when I returned after the long hours away, and without whose love, support and guidance over many years my work on this book would not have been possible. Also to my father, Professor Kenneth Kirby, who died prematurely aged 49 from heart disease, whose dedication and inspiration have been a motivating force for me over the years.

It has been both an honour and a pleasure to work with Victoria, whose enthusiasm and motivation is infectious. We hope this book will transform the lives of many people who don't know where or how to ask difficult questions about one of the most important strands of their lives. We don't know all the answers, but what we and others didn't know, we have tried to discover over the last 26 years. Many of these discoveries lie within this book.

Acknowledgements

A year ago, I received a telephone call asking me to put pen to paper and write this book. I knew I could not write it alone, so I thought of Professor Mike Kirby, whom I admire and respect. I would ask him to help me and together we would write a book which would highlight the importance of intimacy.

He has shown extraordinary patience with me, and I am very proud and still overwhelmed that a man with so many other responsibilities has had the time to meet up with me at every conference, listened to me and replied to all my emails. He is one of those very good men, and I am privileged to have his name by the side of mine. Interestingly, his father also died young and hence we both have an understanding of the importance of good health, the pain of grief, and the need to share our knowledge with others and turn pain and sadness into something good. My son Samuel, whilst standing in the kitchen cooking with me, came up with the wonderful title, "Sleeping with ED." So apologies to anyone called Edward out there and no, it is not at all biographical!

I would love to thank some of the very special friends and family in my life, and colleagues at work who at times of crisis have kept me buoyant and through all the traumas have managed to help me to keep a level head and a smile on my face. So special, thanks go to: Josh Mills, Tracey Cox, Julia and David Montgomery, Jane Head Lee, Carmella Brewer, Tracey Luhr, Martin and Dorothy Farndell, Jan Van de Pol, Edward Hilton, Laura Pritchard, my exceptional good friend and ballroom dance teacher Carol Bolton, who somehow manages to get my head, feet and body working in the right direction after many hours of practice! Also a thank you to the cartoonist, Graham Hagan, who has interpreted our somewhat quirky suggestions with empathy and humour.

A very special depth of gratitude to every single man and woman who has had the courage to attend a session with me; I have been privileged to know you all. Each one of you has trusted me with your most innermost fears about intimacy and relationships and without you this book would never have been written.

Finally my mother who, bless her, as always had some difficulty understanding my job, and still rings me in the week and thinks I don't work, but is probably my greatest friend of all. She is proud of me and loves me very much and having her respect and kindness has made the time alone much easier to manage.

CHAPTER 1

Introduction

It takes two to get it right!

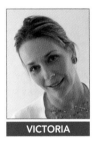

VICTORIA

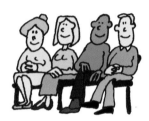

Whether you are sleeping with ED (erectile dysfunction) or waking up in the morning with a partner experiencing ED, this book is for you.

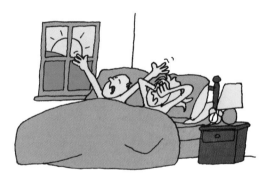

I have spent 20 years working with men and women with sexual problems and I am utterly passionate about the importance of intimacy. When I reached the age of 39, my husband Martin, aged only 48, died suddenly of a heart attack. He had not been well for many years before, but like many men he refused to go to the doctor. In retrospect I wish I had handcuffed him and dragged him along to have a health check. He could have lived and my three extraordinary children would have had a father. At least it would have helped to have had some warning, but all those years ago we did not have the knowledge that we have now about the dangers of cholesterol and heart disease.

This book is a way of using all my heartache and sadness to ensure that as few men, women, children, and friends as possible, ever have to experience the distress, shock and unhappiness that followed that dreadful day. My children have been just the best, they have made me laugh and cry, but mostly smile.

Lucy used to tell her teachers at school that I could tell what sexual problems they had just by shaking their hands; I always wondered why at school meetings, so few teachers wanted to welcome me!

Samuel asked me one day to remove a vibrator from the fruit bowl as he had a new girlfriend coming round. I obviously had been lecturing the night before and was showing a variety of sex toys to the audience. Like a good mother, I returned home and placed it safely in my office, only to find out the next morning that two vibrators were charging up outside his bedroom door! Sam left me a message: "Thank you for taking the vibrators from the fruit bowl but you left two charging up outside my bedroom door. My girlfriend was not impressed! She says that most families charge up mobile phones."

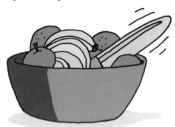

Every day when I wake up, I am delighted to be able to go to work. I know that I shall have the privilege of meeting men and women who are worried about some aspect of their sex life and the effect that it has had on their relationship.

I believe that everyone deserves a hug, without feeling anxious that they will be expected to continue with some further intimacy. That's the problem with erectile dysfunction or any sexual problem. When a penis loses its erection or ejaculation happens to early or too slowly, or a partner experiences pain on intercourse, the brain logs the response very quickly. Then as soon as any intimacy begins, the brain says "stop - hang on. The last time you did this it didn't go very well, you were unhappy and your partner was anxious, so don't try it again." And so just one hug can lead to variety of overwhelming feelings and in the end, relationship resentments.

I am not convinced that intercourse is what we should all be striving for, but I am convinced that everyone deserves to have at least the opportunity to be able to hold someone close to them, to be able to touch their hands, to touch one another, to have a kiss without experiencing fear, and to have someone lie next to them feeling warm and comforted.

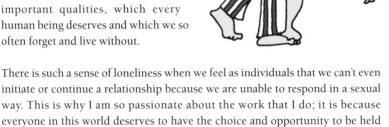

After my husband died, I remember standing on a railway station and being handed a cup of tea. The man's fingers touched mine. I felt this warm feeling throughout my body, skin to skin, he smiled. These are all such important qualities, which every human being deserves and which we so often forget and live without.

There is such a sense of loneliness when we feel as individuals that we can't even initiate or continue a relationship because we are unable to respond in a sexual way. This is why I am so passionate about the work that I do; it is because everyone in this world deserves to have the choice and opportunity to be held closely by another.

When I first started training as a sex therapist, most sexual problems were thought to be psychological, all in the mind, but now we know so much more. Over 70% of sexual problems can have a cause that is physical. Of course, the physical causes may improve, but the psychological worries about being able to perform remain and that is why my work with patients has been such a rewarding and privileged journey.

There are many books about enhancing your sex life, but so little about the effects that medications, illness, surgery and depression have on sexual response, not only on us but also on our partners. It is time to address these issues. We are living longer, and that means we 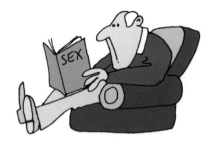 will all need to adapt to changing life styles and address health concerns. Let us start by having a greater depth of understanding, talking openly and honestly with one another, but most of all respecting each other's difficulties and being kind and considerate.

I implore every one of you reading this book not to panic when you or your partner or you experience a sexual problem. There is an answer out there, your doctor will listen, he will examine you and send you for tests and you will get better and learn to cope with the difficulty.

I want to stop everyone putting their heads in the sand like ostriches and thinking that the problem will go away. Intimacy and physical closeness is too important to walk away from. The longer we don't deal with problems, the bigger they become. Imagine a ball of wool in one colour only. When your partner gets involved it becomes two colours and as time passes and the problem continues it becomes multicoloured. Then each strand will have to be unravelled, examined

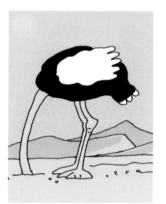 and dealt with separately. If we manage a problem as soon as it begins, we stop the problem contaminating so many other areas of our lives.

I hope you enjoy the book. All I have wanted to achieve is to highlight the link between medical illness, medication, and surgery and show how our relationships and sexual activity can be altered when we have to face difficult times in our lives. So many books are written for health professionals but this book is just for you.

MIKE

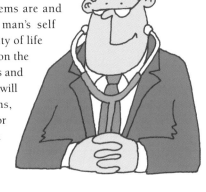

As a practicing physician for over 30 years, I have become aware of how common erectile problems are and how detrimental to a man's self esteem and overall quality of life they can be. The impact on the man and the partner can be enormous and may be deeply traumatising. Many men will admit to occasional erectile problems, often precipitated by the use of alcohol or when they are stressed or tired, but a significant number will admit to a persistent problem.

Erectile dysfunction (ED) is often attributed to the inevitable consequence of aging and although there are significant changes in the aging man, many men lead a happy and fulfilling sex life well into their 80s, when they have a willing partner. The availability of new and effective therapies has made it possible for this extremely common medical condition to be increasingly understood and managed in primary care and there is a solution to the problem for almost everyone.

What has surprised me over the years is how long it takes for the majority of men to 'get around to talking about it'. There are many barriers and this book will focus on how they can be overcome. In the majority of cases, particularly in older men, there is a physical cause for the ED and it is a symptom not a diagnosis. The most common physical causes of ED are conditions that reduce arterial blood flow to the erectile tissues or conditions that damage the nervous system, such as hardening of the arteries, high blood pressure or diabetes.

ED may often be the first presenting symptom of previously undiagnosed medical conditions and it is important for both patients and health professionals to be proactive in the identification of ED. This will not only help restore a normal sexual relationship but also enable underlying diseases to be diagnosed at an earlier stage.

Sex is a very important part of our daily lives. During adolescence, boys compete to lose their virginity; young men judge themselves on the size, firmness and staying power of their erections and their number of sexual partners, and older men may worry about not being able to achieve an erection at all.

The ability to attain and maintain an erection is integral to a man's sense of wellbeing and can be crucial in maintaining a good relationship with his partner. An inability to 'perform' poses a direct threat to a man's core belief in himself. Although it's normal for sexual interest and capacity to decline with advancing age, it becomes an issue when it is not proportional to the needs of the man or his partner. More than 80% of men and 60% of women up to the age of 80 years feel that sex is an important part of their lives and at least 57% of men and 51% of women of middle age still have sex regularly one or more times a week. Embarrassment, fear and ignorance can result in a significant number of men failing to discuss the problem with a health professional and often their partner as well.

In three out of four relationships, the man will initiate the sexual activity, but once ED becomes established the man may with withdraw from sexual activity completely, fearing that he may be unable to 'perform'. The end result of this is failure to have any form of contact that could be seen as a prelude to sex. This can place a huge strain on a relationship, as neither partner is now receiving any form of affection or physical contact.

We hope that this book will be the first step for many men and women in helping them to identify the problem, manage the problem and restore a satisfying sexual relationship.

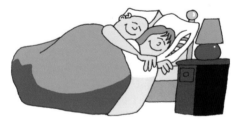

The term impotence (traditionally applied to erection difficulties) is derived from the Latin for 'loss of power'. This association with a lack of strength and vigour automatically connects the condition with the opposite of all that we consider masculine. For centuries men have linked their self respect to the performance of their penis. Therefore, when their penis fails them they no longer feel like a 'real man'. However, ED is extremely common and because the word 'impotence' was considered derogatory, the term erectile dysfunction (ED) was coined.

ED is defined as the inability to achieve or maintain an erection sufficient for sexual activity. It can occur for both physical and psychological reasons and this is because there is a complex interaction between a number of psychological and physical factors necessary for an erection to occur.

If you or your partner have ED, then you are not alone – up to 52% of men between the ages of 40 and 70 years will have experienced some degree of ED and of course, it is age related, occurring in somewhere around 39% of men aged 40 years and rising to around 67% among those aged 70 and over.

Night time and spontaneous day time erections is a sign of good health and tell us important things about both the blood flow and the nerve supply to the penis. To be able to understand why ED occurs it is necessary to review the basic structure of the penis, which is a vascular organ divided into three cylinders, known as the corpora cavernosa and the corpus spongeosum. The paired corpora cavernosa, which constitutes the bulk of the penis, are surrounded by a thick fibrous sheath which supports the rigidity of erectile function. The corpus spongeosum surrounds the urethra, which is the tube that passes out of the bladder down the penis to the exterior, and the corpus spongeosum expands to form the glans of the penis.

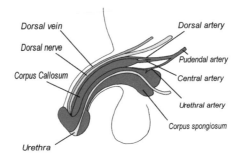

There are two important factors necessary to achieve an erection. One is a good and healthy blood supply and the second a healthy nervous system. Erections are good for erections, which is why the night time erections occur in healthy men. Most men without erectile problems experience on average between four and six erections each night lasting about 100 minutes in total duration and mostly associated with rapid eye movement (REM) sleep. It is thought the purpose of this is to provide increased oxygen to the penile tissues which keep it healthy.

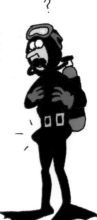

Erection

In response to sexual stimulation, which may be with or without tactile stimulation of the penis, the nervous system causes blood vessels in the penis to fill with blood and at the same time the muscle within the penis relaxes, allowing the flow of blood into the corpora cavernosa, resulting in a rigid erection. The erection hardness scale (EHS) is a simple test of your erection and there is no doubt that achieving a four is better than a three. See Table 1.1 below.

Table 1.1: Erection Hardness Grading Scale (EHGS)

Grade 1	Grade 2	Grade 3	Grade 4
Penis is larger but not hard	Penis is hard but not hard enough for penetration	Penis is hard enough for penetration but not completely hard	Penis is completely hard and fully rigid

When the erotic stimulus has stopped or ejaculation has occurred, detumescense (flaccidity) occurs due to a reduction in blood flow into the penis and contraction of the muscle which allows blood to flow out of the organ.

Health professionals use a series of questions to try and discover whether the ED is due to psychological or physical causes.

Table 1.2: Distinguishing between psychological and physical causes of ED[1]

Psychological	Physical
▪ Sudden onset	▪ Gradual onset
▪ Specific situation	▪ All circumstances
▪ Normal nocturnal and early morning erections	▪ Absent nocturnal and early morning erections
▪ Relationship problems	▪ Normal libido and ejaculation
▪ Problems during sexual development	▪ Normal sexual development

Table 1.3: Distinguishing between psychological and physical causes of ED[1]

Possible psychological causes of ED
▪ Anxiety or stress due to work, personal or finance related matters
▪ Psychological trauma or abuse
▪ Anxiety about sexual performance or sexual identity
▪ Sexual problems in the partner
▪ Relationship/intimacy problems
▪ Depression
▪ Psychosis
▪ Misconceptions/lack of sex education

There are many physical causes of ED, illustrated in Figure 1.1 below.

Figure 1.1:
Physical causes of ED

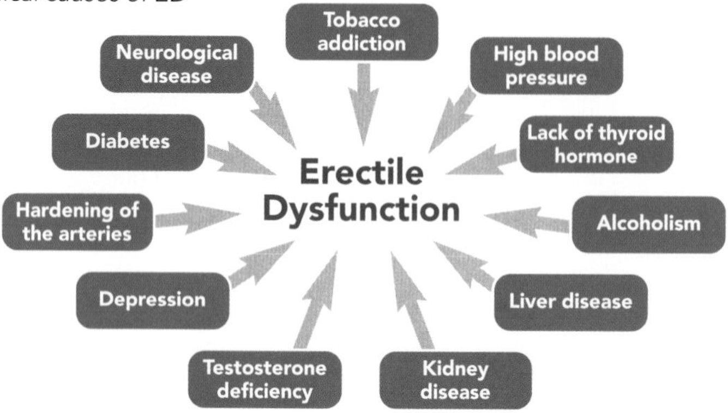

So who is at risk?

Cardiac disease and ED share many risk factors and the early detection of ED gives us time to address these risk factors which may well prevent eventual cardiovascular disease such as a heart attack or stroke.

Table 1.4: Risk factors for cardiovascular disease and their incidence in the UK[2]

Risk factor	Incidence in men	Incidence in women
Overweight / Obesity	46% overweight Further 17% obese	32% overweight Further 21% obese
Raised blood pressure	41%	33%
Raised blood cholesterol	66%	67%
Diabetes	3%	3%
Smoking	28%	26%
Alcohol consumption over daily recommended amounts	38%	21%
Physical activity less than 30 minutes on five days per week	63%	75%

CHAPTER 2

Talking about it

VICTORIA

Why don't men talk about it?

Why is it so difficult for men to talk about a sexual problem, particularly impotence or ejaculation concerns? Most men would say that they are terribly embarrassed and distressed that they are unable to fulfil their partner's needs. Some men believe that if they talk about the problem it will get worse, and if they leave intimacy out of the relationship for a while the next time everything will be fine.

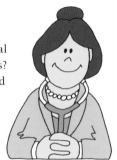

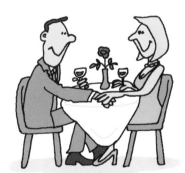

Men on average still wait up to two to three years before visiting their doctor about a sexual problem. The reason for this is mainly embarrassment, but it is also a fear that the doctor might find something seriously wrong with their general health.

I wonder whether women find it easier because we are often asked by our doctors about contraception and our menstrual cycles. We also undergo vaginal examinations, which gives us the opportunity to talk about sexual problems. However, I don't think any of

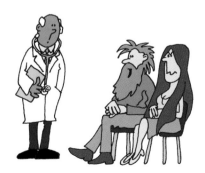

us find it very easy to talk about lack of desire or boredom in the bedroom. Men are very different creatures to us; they aren't comfortable with telling their friends that they couldn't get an erection last night or that they ejaculated prematurely. It seems that a male sexual problem is rarely shared with other men, whereas many women will talk to their friends about difficulties without feeling they are losing their womanhood. It seems that men just don't feel masculine if they are unable to maintain an erection.

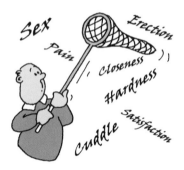

Imagine the scenario: foreplay is all going well and then at the moment of penetration or even when you are getting into position for penetration the erection subsides. What happens next is common for most couples. You either try to stuff the soft penis into the vagina hoping that it will revive the erection, or you stop being sexual for a while and then try and go back to where you left off. Most of the time there is a deadly silence, both partners roll over, we eventually fall asleep and another day dawns.

I think it is time that men were helped to talk about this very sensitive and distressing event. First of all, we need to find the right language; but what words do we use? I think that women often avoid talking to our partners about a sexual problem because they are afraid to hear that the reason they have lost the erection may be due to us. We are frightened that our partners no longer find us attractive or our vaginas are not tight enough, so that the stimulation is not sufficient. How could we ever compete with a man's hand!

We take love making far too seriously, sadly, and unless we talk we will never find a way of resolving the problems.

How to talk about it

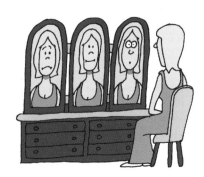

They say that the reason women may appear to be critical is because they are craving intimacy. In fact, men and women have many different ways of communicating.

There are so many social constructs and assumptions surrounding communication – the use of silence, the sound of the voice, our facial expressions and the use of words, that it is no wonder we have difficulty in expressing ourselves at times. In a relationship it is important to respect each other's views and to empathise with one another, but we are often in such a rush to get our point of view across that we don't really listen to what the other person is saying. The key is to take the discussion slowly and speak calmly about our fears and anxieties.

If you are having difficulty here are some suggestions:

Set aside a period of time to talk with no interruptions. Take the phone off the hook, put the animals outside, close the door and decide what you will do if the door bell rings. You will need to agree on the time and not just grab your partner to sit down at the last minute.

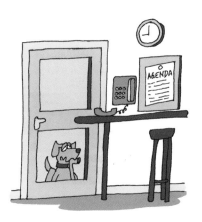

You need to agree on an agenda, whether writing things down before you come to the 'talk time', or setting aside five minutes prior to speaking, to agree on a subject each that you feel needs discussing.

You also need to agree on the amount of time you are setting aside. I would suggest a maximum of half an hour. If you don't do this the talking will never end, and there always needs to be a beginning (the agenda), a middle (discussion) and an end (understanding and agreement).

One of you needs to begin speaking for 10 minutes; try and stay focused and define the problem. It helps to sit without your arms and legs crossed or curled up on a seat; it's amazing how much more adult our conversations are when we put both feet on the ground, our hands by our side and our head is held up.

When one has finished talking ask your partner to summarise what you have said. One of the reasons we never seem to resolve important issues is because we feel that we have not been heard. Women especially need a sign that the information has been received. If your partner summarises well, that's fine, but if it still seems unclear, you may need to repeat some of what you have said and try again, until you are sure you have been understood.

The next stage is to ask your partner to talk about their anxieties and again repeat back to them what was said. Finally, you switch again and ask for what you would like, and what would have to happen for the issue to be resolved. Each time, the partner paraphrases what the other has said.

Always try and use the word "I" and own your problems, rather than saying "you" or "we". It makes our thoughts and feelings personal and stops the other person feeling that they are to blame for everything. The other words which seem at times unhelpful are "should" or "ought".

At the end of the time together, be kind to one another. If it is appropriate, give one another a hug, or make a cup of tea. Whenever I do something a little different and difficult, I always spoil myself afterwards with a chocolate cake, or I may even buy myself some flowers.

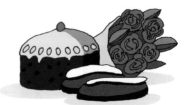

REFERENCES
1. Impotence Association Survey, 2000-2002
2. www.lovelifematters.co.uk

CHAPTER 3

So does your partner have diabetes?

MIKE

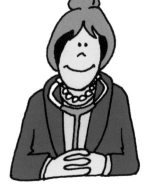

Understanding diabetes

If you or your partner have already been diagnosed with diabetes, your doctor or nurse will have explained that it occurs when the amount of glucose (sugar) in the blood is too high because the body cannot produce enough of the hormone called insulin to help convert the glucose into 'essential fuel for the body'.

There are two main types of diabetes:

- **Type 1** (insulin dependent diabetes, when the body cannot make insulin at all)
- **Type 2** (when the pancreas gland makes too little insulin and when the body becomes resistant to the effects of insulin)

Type 1 diabetes always requires insulin therapy. Type 2 diabetes is normally treated with tablets, but eventually many patients with this disease will also need to use additional insulin by injection. The treatments for diabetes aim to keep the glucose, blood pressure and cholesterol levels in the body as close to normal as possible. A healthy lifestyle, together with regular medical treatment for diabetes will help to keep the body healthy and avoid longer term problems with nerves, arteries, heart, kidneys, eyes and feet, together with normal sexual function.

Figure 3.1: *Chronic Complications of Diabetes*
(The Audit Commission. Testing Times. A Review of Diabetes Services in England and Wales, 2000)

Chronic Complications of Diabetes

Retinopathy
Most common cause of blindness in people of working age

Nephropathy
16% of all new patients needing renal replacement therapy

Erectile Dysfunction
May affect up to 50% of men with long standing diabetes

Coronary and Cerebrovascular Disease
2 – 4 fold increase risk of coronary heart disease and stroke; 75% have hypertension

Foot Problems
15% of people with diabetes develop foot ulcers; 5 – 15% of people with diabetic foot ulcers need amputations

Common signs of undiagnosed or poorly controlled diabetes are increased thirst, having to pass urine more often, especially at night, tiredness, weight loss and blurred vision. In diabetes, erection problems generally occur due to complications damaging the muscle, arteries or nerves in the penis. In Type 1 diabetes this is usually some years after the diabetes has been detected and diagnosed. Type 2 diabetes on the other hand, can often go undetected for many years and complications, including ED, may be a warning sign for previously undetected or undiagnosed diabetes. ED can also be a warning sign of undetected heart and circulation disease.

Of course, problems with erections or your sex life may not be due to the physical effects of diabetes at all and it may be just the worry over your diabetes that is affecting your sex life generally. As many as one in four men with diabetes may have erection problems because of emotional factors rather than a physical cause. Having diabetes doesn't automatically mean that men will have problems with erections or sex life generally. However, if any changes are noticed in the quality of the erections, then try not to be embarrassed to talk to your doctor or nurse – they are there to help you and there are good treatments available. If you have diabetes it is very important not to smoke, since this greatly increases the risk of complications.

ED can be an early warning sign of diabetes and we know that in the UK there are approximately 1 million people who have diabetes but don't know they have it. Early detection is important because diabetic tendency can exist for up to 10 years before symptoms develop and during this time damage can be done to the health of the blood vessels and nerves. A fasting blood glucose test is a routine investigation when men present with ED. Early detection of diabetes is also important because good management of the condition prevents complications.

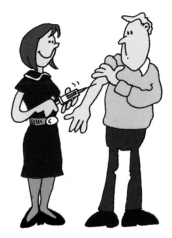

Middle aged men with diabetes are around five times more likely to be affected by cardiovascular disease than men without diabetes. The condition is associated with being overweight and the incidence of diabetes has increased by around two-thirds in men since the early 1990s. There are currently about 1.4 million people in the UK diagnosed with diabetes.

The cardiovascular and neurological complications associated with diabetes increase the risk of ED by a very complex mechanism. They interfere with the interaction between the vascular endothelium (lining of the blood vessel walls) and the smooth muscle cells in the penis. Over 50% of men with diabetes have suffered with ED at some time and as many as 39% suffer with ED all the time. The onset of ED in diabetic men usually occurs gradually and often 10-15 years earlier than those without diabetes. There is a striking degree of overlap between the typical problems associated with diabetes and risk factors for ED, including:

- Peripheral neuropathy (disease of the nerves outside of the brain and spinal cord)
- Vascular insufficiency (insufficient blood supply to the penis)
- Dysfunction of the cavernosal endothelium (lining of the blood vessel walls) and smooth muscle
- Poor blood glucose control
- Treated or untreated high blood pressure
- Low testosterone levels
- Obesity
- History of smoking

The greater the length of time a man has diabetes, and the quality of glucose control, determines the risk of ED. In addition to this, poor control of diabetes makes ED more difficult to treat.

VICTORIA

The chances are that your partner has probably developed diabetes in later life and therefore has the Type 2 variety. Type 1 diabetes tends to develop at a young age and Type 2 often develops in middle or later life. Type 2 is often treated with oral tablets, diet and exercise.

It is so important that men with unpredictable ED go to their doctor and have a urine check for sugar or have a blood test. Also, free treatment is available for erection problems if you have diabetes.

Men with diabetes often have some high blood pressure problems and the nerves often do not send strong enough signals; this will interfere with the erection response, not just because of the tablets which are often prescribed, but because of the damage to tissue inside the penis, which means that the blood flow isn't as effective as it could be.

So, clearly, there are a few complications which need to be taken into account along with diabetes, especially if you are intending to have a satisfactory sex life. Some men are also obese, which makes particular sexual positions uncomfortable.

The problem with some illnesses is that you can often become such a good nurse when looking after your partner, making sure that his diet is good, that he is exercising, and going to his clinic check-ups and being generally worried about his health, that no one seems to be looking after you and recognising the important part you have to play. How many times have you been at a consultation with your partner and the doctor asks: "How are YOU coping"!

Wouldn't it be lovely if sometimes health professionals, friends and family realised that although our partners are ill, we are also being great carers and would like some recognition – after all, just because they need so much attention doesn't mean that we don't need any either! We can feel quite cross if our partners don't say thank you occasionally, which can lead to resentment – not conducive to intimacy.

When we look after someone in a relationship because they are ill, we often lose our interest in sexual activity because the roles have changed; after all, nurses don't have sex with their patients, so we need to be particularly aware of this and discuss the changes with our partners. Please never be afraid to ask a doctor what the side effects might be with certain treatments for diabetes.

So let's look at the changes that occur to the erections of those men with diabetes. First of all you tend to notice that the penis is just not as hard as it used to be during foreplay, and when intercourse occurs it seems to 'go down' after a short while. When men realise this they tend to shorten foreplay, because they think they are going to lose their erection, so best get it in before it goes away! We can often be tempted to think: "He hasn't paid much attention to my needs and is just thinking about himself. So the next time he wants sex I'll avoid it and make him pay"!

Some men notice that their orgasm sensations change: either it feels a little numb and not as powerful as before, or the ejaculation fluid can go back into the bladder. This can happen in about 50% of diabetic men. These men do orgasm, it's just that nothing comes out, and we all get a bit confused as to whether there has been an ending or not. The man can tell if this happens because when he next passes urine, it will often be cloudy. Some men ejaculate quickly because they are anxious about losing their erection and some have delayed ejaculation, so expect some changes and don't panic – just ask your doctor and talk about it together.

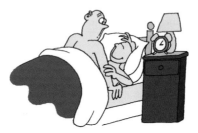

Now, if your partner has diabetes he will probably need to use some treatments to help maintain his erections. He might have reduced hormone levels too, so his urge to have sex may also be a little less than before.

There are a variety of treatments available such as the oral drugs like Viagra (Sildenafil), Levitra (Vardenafil), and Cialis (Tadalafil), as well as injection therapy and vacuum therapy. Often a combination of these is used. Whichever one you choose, it is far better if it is a joint decision, so make sure you attend the consultation with your partner and talk about the advantages and disadvantages of each treatment.

CASE STUDY 1

John was 52, overweight and feeling tired and thirsty. Mary, his wife, was worried about his tiredness and made an appointment for him to see the doctor. They had not been having intercourse for about a year, because John's erections had not lasted long enough for pleasurable intercourse.

John had some tests which showed sugar in his urine and was diagnosed with Type 2 diabetes. He was instructed to change his diet and use tablets to control his blood sugar levels.

As the lack of a good erection had been a concern to them, they told their doctor that their love life had diminished. Their doctor prescribed an oral tablet. John initially used it with masturbation to get used to the drug. When he felt confident, Mary and he increased foreplay and were able to enjoy a more pleasurable and enjoyable sex life. They also recognised the importance of looking after their health and started walking out together in the evenings, always holding hands!

CASE STUDY 2

Howard had developed diabetes as a young man, and had got used to diabetic clinics and making sure that he measured his blood sugar levels regularly. He used insulin injections to control his blood sugar. He explained his Type 1 diabetes to his partner, Julie, and the long term consequences.

Both agreed it would be helpful if Julie joined him at the clinic appointments. Howard had at times found it difficult to ejaculate and his erections were sometimes unpredictable. Julie had thought that this was all her fault and was worried about their relationship. They decided to have some couple counselling to talk about Julie's anxiety and also discuss the variety of treatments that were available to them.

TOP TIPS

It is very important that if you have diabetes and ED, you pay particular attention to the following:

- A twice daily exercise regime such as 20 minutes brisk walking on at least five days per week
- Careful control of your diet
- Try to lose any excess weight
- Keep fit for sex by indulging regularly
- Take the medication reliably
- Attend for regular check-ups
- Know your own numbers, eg blood pressure, HbA1c (which tells us how good your glucose control has been over the last three months) and cholesterol
- Don't be embarrassed to tell your doctor that your partner is having erection problems
- Talk to your partner about the erection changes you have noticed
- Share the decision making about treatments
- Increase foreplay and direct stimulation to the genitals
- Use a lubricant on the penis to enhance stimulation
- Have sex in "daylight hours" when neither of you is too tired

MIKE

Neurological causes of ED

Any disease process or injury affecting the brain, spinal cord or pelvic nerves can cause ED. In some cases the erectile problems are just one of the multiple disabilities caused by widespread disease within the central nervous system. These disabilities may impinge on sexual function in a number of ways, all of which need to be considered when planning therapy.

Spinal cord injury is a condition which commonly affects young men and can cause ED. With complete high spinal cord lesions, psychogenic erections do not occur, although many men may show reflex erections in response to genital stimulation. With complete lower spinal cord injuries, there is often associated damage to the blood supply and these reflex erections are lost. Incomplete spinal cord injuries produce a more variable pattern, as do diseases of the spinal cord such as multiple sclerosis.

If the nerves are damaged, the oral medications do not work effectively, but injection therapy may be helpful. However, in the case of neurogenic ED, only very small doses of Caverjet (Alprostadil) are necessary, as this group are often very sensitive to these compounds and therefore at considerable risk of developing a prolonged erection.

CASE STUDY 3

Tom was involved in a road traffic accident that damaged his spine; from the waist down nothing worked as before and tablets prescribed for ED were not helpful. Tom was seen by a specialist who taught him how to inject his penis using a special device, which always produced the erection he needed.

CHAPTER 4

My heart aches; cardiac issues

MIKE

Introduction

If your partner has recently had a heart problem, whether it is heart attack or angina, and has needed to see a doctor about his symptoms, there is always that worry that sex will bring on more pain or cause another heart attack.

In fact, research shows that less than 1% of cases of heart attacks are related to sexual activity. There is more likelihood of problems occurring if sex happens with an unfamiliar partner, so if you are in a compatible long-standing relationship and know one another's bodies, problems are very unlikely. Many men and their partners are very anxious about resuming sexual activity. You can, in fact, start thinking about having sex again up to two to three weeks after the event. Sexual activity is not a strenuous activity as long as you talk about your concerns before hand, discuss the matter with your doctor and take things slowly to start with.

ED and cardiovascular disease

ED can occur in as many as 39 – 64% of male patients with cardiovascular disease. Cardiovascular disease (CVD) is caused by hardening of the arteries; a generalised process that involves blood flow to the legs, heart and brain. It is a gradual process that starts in young adulthood and progresses throughout our lives. It is caused by a gradual deposition of cholesterol in the walls of the arteries that causes thickening and narrowing of the blood vessel and eventually compromises the blood flow.

When it involves the blood vessels in the legs, it may cause a condition known as intermittent claudication, which is characterised by pain in the calves on walking and is usually relieved by rest. When it affects the coronary arteries of the heart, it may lead to angina and eventually a heart attack. When it affects the blood vessels to the brain it can cause a stroke or a condition known as transient ischaemic attack (TIA) which is a type of mini-stroke that occurs for a short period of time and then gets better. This is a very important warning sign that should not be ignored.

There are certain conditions that increase the risk of cardiovascular disease and these include:

- High blood pressure
- Diabetes
- High cholesterol
- Overweight
- Obesity
- Lack of exercise or sedentary lifestyle
- A diet high in saturated fat and salt, and low in fruit, vegetables and wholegrains
- Smoking
- Having a family history of heart disease
- Having ED

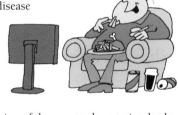

ED can be an early sign of vascular disease. This is because the arteries that supply blood to the penis are very small and endothelial dysfunction, which is the

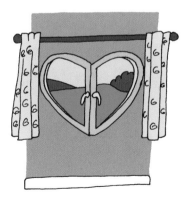

first sign of damage to the arteries, leads to ED. The endothelium is a very thin layer of cells which line all our blood vessels. It is very important to keep this layer of cells healthy by leading a healthy lifestyle. We know that ED can be an early warning sign of cardiovascular disease and it can occur five years before other more significant signs such as angina or a heart attack. Therefore the penis has been described as 'the window to the heart of man'.

Loss of night time erections and spontaneous early morning or day time erections should be an early prompt to attend your doctor's surgery for a check-up. Men with heart disease, diabetes or high blood pressure are up to four times more likely to develop some degree of ED compared with men who do not suffer from these disorders. ED can also tell us about the severity of the coronary artery disease, because those men with the most severe coronary artery disease have the least firm erections. The penis has therefore also been described as the barometer of cardiovascular health.

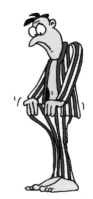

Table 4.1: Artery size and Atherothrombosis
(Montorsi et al, Eur Urol 2003; 44:352-4)

Artery	Size (mm)	Clinical Event
Penile	1 - 2	ED
Coronary	3 - 4	CAD
Carotid	5 - 7	TIA (mini-stroke or stroke)
Femoral	6 - 8	Claudication

High blood pressure

There is a clear link between ED and high blood pressure; in one study in men with high blood pressure, mild ED was found in 7.7%, moderate ED in 15.4% and severe ED in 45.2%. When questioned, 60.9% of men with high blood pressure and 77.9% of men with both high blood pressure and diabetes admitted to ED problems. Many of the tablets prescribed for high blood pressure can cause ED and some are worse than others. If you have high blood pressure and ED, the best choice of drug is likely to be one known as a sartan. This group of drugs for treating high blood pressure are not only less likely to cause ED than all the others, but may also improve the situation.

If you have high blood pressure you need to know your numbers, including cholesterol and blood pressure, and have a regular test for diabetes, especially if you are overweight.

The myth that sex can be dangerous

This has been perpetuated through the media; for example, in 1975 the former US Vice President Nelson Rockefeller died at the age of 70 in the company of his 25-year old personal assistant Megan Marshack. Other famous victims of death during sexual intercourse include Pope Leo VIII in 965 and the former French President Felix Faure in 1899. Incidences such as these give rise to the incorrect assumption that normal sexual activity can be dangerous.

There have no doubt been situations where men have had heart attacks during sexual intercourse; however, the odds of this happening stand at one sudden death per 1.51 million episodes of exertion and, interestingly, research tells us that the majority of sexual activity related sudden deaths usually involve sex with an unfamiliar and often much younger partner, in an unfamiliar setting and after excessive alcohol and food.

After developing heart disease, fears surrounding the safety of resuming or initiating sexual activity can, in some instances, play an important part in the development of ED. In reality, sex is literally a walk in the park and should be regarded as a normal form of exercise, and not necessarily a strenuous one at that. Research tells us that during sex the heart rate rises on average to 120 beats per minute and the blood pressure rises modestly. The duration of sex for older people is normally five to 15 minutes, with the peak physical effect taking place at three to five minutes. Similar changes in pulse and blood pressure occur during a normal working day. Table 4.2 overleaf helps put this into perspective and shows the metabolic equivalent of the task for various daily activities, as well as sexual intercourse.

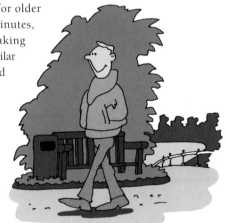

Table 4.2: *Metabolic equivalent of the task (MET)*[3]

Daily activity	MET score rating
Sexual intercourse with an established partner:	
Lower range – 'normal'	2-3
Upper range – 'vigorous activity'	5-6
Lifting and carrying objects (9-20kg)	4-5
Walking one mile in 20 minutes on level ground	3-4
Golf	4-5
Gardening	3-5
DIY, wallpapering, etc.	4-5
Light housework, eg ironing, polishing	2-4
Heavy housework, eg making beds, scrubbing floors	3-6

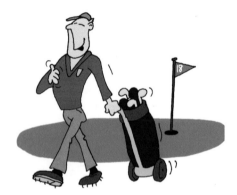

We know that sex does not significantly increase the risk of stroke and that it does offer some protection against a future heart attack. Men having intercourse regularly, up to two times per week, are less likely to have heart disease than men who just have occasional episodes of sex.

Heart attacks can be triggered by exertion, anger and emotion, but often the trigger is unknown. During normal daily life the baseline risk of suffering a heart attack is only one chance in a million per hour for a healthy adult and 10 chances in a million per hour for a patient with known cardiovascular disease.

The risk of triggering a heart attack in a patient with known cardiovascular disease following sex increases only minimally to approximately only 30 chances in a million per hour, compared to 10 chances in a million per hour during normal daily activity. This means that sex is a likely contributor to heart attacks in men with known heart disease in less than 1% of cases. In the long term it is likely that the tension generated by sexual frustration will be more harmful than the excitement generated by sexual intercourse.

Exercise testing

The risk of heart attack is related to overall fitness and general cardiovascular health. One way to evaluate blood flow to the heart is to perform an exercise test, either on an exercise bicycle or on a treadmill. We know that if a man can achieve 5-6 METs (see Table 4.2 regarding MET equivalents), without any change in the ECG, the development of an irregular heart or a fall in blood pressure, they can be reassured that they are not at risk during normal sexual activity.

Exercise tolerance can also be assessed with a simple question: 'Can you walk a mile on the flat in 20 minutes without becoming breathless or developing chest pain?' If you do experience chest pain, shortness of breath or an irregular heartbeat during this type of activity this does warrant further investigation.

CVD patients at low risk of suffering a heart attack from sexual activity

Such patients can usually be sexually active and receive treatment for ED safely. They include the following:

Asymptomatic patients (symptom free with less than three risk factors for cardiovascular disease)
- Patients are at low risk of any significant cardiac complications from sexual activity or treatment of ED

Patients with hypertension (high blood pressure) which is controlled with medication
- These patients can safely receive ED treatments
- However, antihypertensive medications may cause ED

Patients with mild stable angina
- If the angina has been evaluated and treated effectively the patient is usually capable of sexual activity
- In patients on the verge of more severe angina, medication may be required to prevent symptoms of shortness of breath or chest pain during sexual activity
- The risk of a heart attack appears to be no greater in these patients than those without cardiovascular disease

Patients who have had a coronary artery bypass graft (CABG) or coronary artery intervention such as angioplasty or stenting
- The risk during sexual activity will depend on the success of the procedure
- Exercise stress testing may help evaluate the degree of treatment success and thus safety for sex; if the procedure is successful, the patient is at low risk

Patients who have had a heart attack (MI) six to eight weeks previously
- Resuming sexual activity after a heart attack is usually safe following a six to eight week recovery period
- Start off with gentle kissing and caressing and as health and confidence grow, resume normal sexual activities
- Taking regular exercise will make you fitter for sex

Patients with mild mitral valve disease
- Patients not at greatly increased risk of cardiac events during sex

Mild congestive heart failure (Class 1)
- This is cardiac disease that allows ordinary physical activities without symptoms and these patients appear to have no increased risk of suffering a cardiac event from sex

CVD patients at intermediate risk of suffering a heart attack from sexual activity

These patients should not attempt to resume sexual activity or undergo treatment for ED until their cardiac health has been re-evaluated. These include the following:

Asymptomatic patients (symptom free but with more than three risk factors for cardiovascular disease)
- These patients may be identified by their GP for having, for example, a sedentary lifestyle, being overweight or obese, smoking etc.

Patients with moderate stable angina
- Symptoms are usually reproducible on exercise testing which may be helpful in predicting risk from sexual activity

Patients who have had a heart attack (MI) two to four weeks previously
- These patients are thought to be at slightly increased risk from sexual activity, which can be assessed with exercise testing

Patients with left ventricular dysfunction / congestive heart failure (Class II)
- These patients are often limited in activities such as walking by shortness of breath and may be at increased risk of a cardiac event from sexual activity
- Assessment, treatment and exercise regime may allow reclassification to a lower risk category and restore confidence in resuming sexual activity

Patients with atherosclerotic disease (hardening of the arteries)
- Patients with disease of the arteries supplying the legs and those who have already had a stroke or transient ischaemic attack (TIA) are thought to be at increased risk of a heart attack and should be considered for cardiac assessment

CVD patients at high risk of suffering a heart attack from sexual activity

Patients defined as those whose cardiac problem is sufficiently severe that sexual activity may be a risk. ED in these patients should not be managed in primary care (by their GP), but should undergo further cardiac assessment by a specialist. Sexual activity should be avoided until either the condition has been stabilised with treatment or the cardiologist has decided that sexual activity may be safely resumed. This group of patients includes those with the following:

Unstable refractory angina
- Angina that is of recent onset, is severe, or occurs at rest
- These patients suffer symptoms on mild exertion

Uncontrolled hypertension (high blood pressure)
- Patients who have high blood pressure that is not controlled with medication, or who have more severe forms of the disease

Congestive heart failure (Class III or IV)
- Characterised by breathlessness when at rest
- These patients are limited by their symptoms, which are provoked easily, such as by walking on the flat

Some types of arrhythmias (abnormal or irregular heart beats)
- Symptoms may include palpitations (racing or fluttering of the heart), breathlessness and chest pain
- These patients can be fitted with a portable ECG machine (Holter monitor) during sexual activity to assess their risk
- Patients with implanted pacemakers or defibrillators are not considered at increased risk of a cardiovascular event from sexual activity.

Moderate to severe heart valve disease (especially aortic stenosis)
- These conditions may restrict the flow of blood through the heart and may cause breathlessness, chest pain or fainting on exertion

Table 4.3: Summary of risk to CVD patients of sexual activity

Risk	Type of patient
Low	■ Asymptomatic patients (symptom free with less than three risk factors for CVD)
	■ Hypertension (high blood pressure) controlled with medication
	■ Patients with mild stable angina
	■ Coronary artery bypass graft or coronary artery intervention (angioplasty or stenting)
	■ Heart attack (MI) six to eight weeks previously
	■ Mild mitral valve disease
	■ Mild congestive heart failure (Class 1)
Medium	■ Asymptomatic patients (symptom free but with more than three risk factors for cardiovascular disease
	■ Patients with moderate stable angina
	■ Patients who have had a heart attack (MI) two to four weeks previously
	■ Patients with left ventricular dysfunction / congestive heart failure (Class II)
	■ Patients with atherosclerotic disease (hardening of the arteries)
High	■ Unstable refractory angina
	■ Uncontrolled hypertension (high blood pressure)
	■ Congestive heart failure (Class III or IV)
	■ Some types of arrhythmias (abnormal or irregular heart beats)
	■ Moderate to severe heart valve disease (especially aortic stenosis)

There is no evidence that any form of ED therapy increases cardiac risk, assuming all the manufacturer's instructions are followed. Sexual intercourse is no more stressful to the heart than many other daily activities.

Getting fit for sex

If ever there was a reason to start a fitness programme, then this is it. Although the risk of having a heart attack during sex is very low, regular physical activity further reduces the risk considerably and also keeps your vascular endothelium healthy. Exercise can also lower the risk of stroke which is probably because regular exercise reduces the risk of high blood pressure, being overweight, and diabetes.

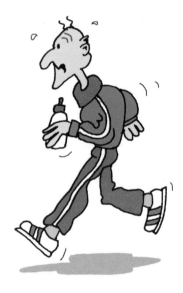

Points to remember

- Don't expect instant success; often up to 12 doses of the drugs for treating ED are needed to re-establish normal erections
- Sexual stimulation is always required because the medication works via the normal processes, so involve your partner
- Attend for regular follow-up
- Report any problems
- Lead a healthy lifestyle

TOP TIPS

If you have ED and cardiovascular disease, the key messages are:

- Take regular exercise – at least 20 minutes twice per day on at least five days per week
- Know your numbers – cholesterol, blood pressure, glucose if you have diabetes
- Eat a healthy diet, low in saturated fat & salt and high in fruit, vegetables and whole grains
- Keep weight under control
- Take your medication regularly
- Keep fit for sex!

If you are prescribed tablets to treat your ED, eg Viagra, Vardenafil or Cialis, these should not be taken with nitrate therapy, eg TNT spray or tablets under the tongue, known as Trinitrin.

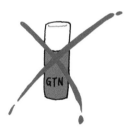

So let's summarize our thoughts on sex and the heart

Men with heart disease, high blood pressure or atherosclerosis (narrowed arteries) may notice a slow but continuing change in being able to achieve or maintain an erection. The same processes that cause heart disease or linked conditions, also affects the penis. When arteries in the general circulation become blocked, this restricts blood flow to the heart and can cause heart disease. When arteries in the penis become blocked, blood flow to the penis is restricted and ED will occur. Don't ignore these changes, talk to your doctor or practice nurse about it.

In general, morning and night time erections without any form of sexual encouragement are a sign of everything working normally. When these types of erections disappear it is important to discuss this with your doctor or nurse.

Lifetime events such as redundancy, divorce, bereavement or a surgical operation can cause ED. This is often related to the emotional feelings at the time. Morning and night time erections usually still occur and the problem may be intermittent. In such cases counselling can be very helpful.

Drinking too much alcohol combined with stress, anxiety or loss of confidence can be the cause of occasional erection problems. However, a poor lifestyle, the consumption of an unhealthy diet, smoking, recreational drug use and lack of exercise are very common causes of erection problems.

If you take regular physical exercise you reduce your risk of a heart attack by at least a half. In the general population there is a very small risk that sexual activity will be the trigger for a heart attack. Having sex uses a similar amount of energy as:

- Walking briskly for 20 minutes on the flat
- Walking for 15 minutes on the flat and up one flight of stairs (20)

It helps to get fit for sex. Sex is no more stressful to the heart than other activities such as playing golf or carrying heavy shopping home. After a heart attack, men and their partners often worry about the safety of returning to sexual activity and, of course, everyone does daily activities with different amounts of energy. The amount of exertion depends on whether you are with a new or an established partner, and after a heart attack it is wise to discuss with your doctor the resumption of sexual activity. Anyone who can manage three to four minutes on a treadmill without getting breathless or experiencing palpitations or chest pain, can usually be reassured that it is safe to have sex.

Victoria talks about sex and the heart

VICTORIA

Of course, during sexual activity the heart rate and blood pressure rises and we use more oxygen. At orgasm they are at their highest and then they decline slowly, but sex in a long standing relationship does not put undue stress on the heart.

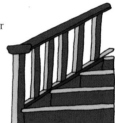

If you imagine the heart beat rises to about 120 beats per minute at orgasm, although this might sound a bit high it is only equal to climbing two flights of stairs fairly quickly. So all you have to do is take your partner to the bottom of a flight of stairs either at the hospital if you are worried, or at home, and watch him climb. If he experiences no pain then he is ready to have sex.

Now of course sexual positions are important here too, so this is where you need to talk to one another. If he has always been used to being on top of you (the 'missionary' position), then I would suggest that you swap places so that you perform most of the movements and he does less of the thrusting. I know it can

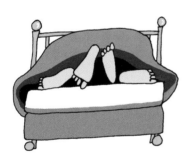

be a little strange at the beginning, but you will be surprised how rewarding it is to be a bit more creative. Many women worry that their partner will see more of their body and especially their breasts. If you feel like this, don't panic, buy yourself a pretty negligee and wear it until you feel more comfortable. It is better to restart intimacy as soon as possible than delay it because you have concerns about your body image.

When men have heart problems, like high blood pressure, they are often prescribed medicine to help. You will probably realise that a few years before the heart attack or heart disease was recognised, your partner was beginning to experience some difficulties in either getting or maintaining an erection. That is why it is so important to talk about sexual problems; as I have said before, an erection problem can be a marker for other health problems.

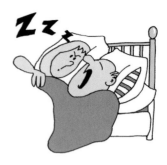

In the early stages of ED you have probably had intermittent good sex; in other words, sometimes the erections have been OK and at other times disastrous. Many of my clients say it is at this time that they start to be less intimate with one another, especially if he has started snoring as well! How useful those spare bedrooms are at this point. He moves out so you can sleep undisturbed. This is one of the worst scenarios, because before you know it, both of you are living separate lives, no more morning cuddles, and even those special talks that you have at night, pass by.

CASE STUDY 4

John was 45, and had a sudden heart attack; no one in the family expected it, even though he had been complaining of some chest pain for a short while. Unfortunately, like many men, he very rarely visited the doctor. The family, especially his partner Jenny, was distraught and very worried.

They were so pleased to have him home after being in hospital that neither of them had talked about if and when they should resume having sex. Months passed and neither said very much; they had a few cuddles in bed but when any touch became slightly sexual both of them withdrew without saying anything to one another. After six months, Jenny noticed that they were not even having a hug before bed and she felt alone and sad that a special part of their relationship had been lost.

Finally, Jenny had the courage to talk to her doctor and he explained that it would be safe for them to resume sex; it was also safe for him to take one of the oral impotence tablets, as there was no contraindication regarding any of John's medication. They started slowly just pleasuring one another, making sure that they increased genital stimulation. Jenny lay on top and they were able to resume having intercourse again. The cuddles and hugs returned.

More TOP TIPS

- If a man can climb briskly two flights of stairs without symptoms – sex will also be symptom free
- If your partner can walk one mile on the flat in 20 minutes without getting breathless or experiencing any chest pain, he is also safe for sex
- If your partner has had surgery on his chest, place a small pillow like the ones you get on airplanes on his chest; this will also help stop any friction on the suture line as well as protect you from the coarse chest hair growing back
- If your partner is on nitrates and gets occasional chest pain, keep the tablets by the side of the bed and use if necessary, but remember never let your partner use an oral impotence drug if he is taking nitrates
- If you are worried, keep a red lipstick by the bed and if he does get any chest pain after taking a tablet for ED and you have to call an ambulance, write the name of the tablet on his forehead, so the paramedics know what treatment to give him safely
- If your partner gets a bit breathless, you may need to take a more active role; in other words it is time to get on top! Increase the foreplay and talk to your doctor
- It is best to have sex in a warm room but NOT within two hours of a heavy meal or a hot bath.
- Sex in the morning is a good idea when you are more relaxed, rather than being tired after a long day

Medication: pills – the good, the bad and the ugly

Medications that can cause ED

MIKE

Many prescription drugs are associated with ED and the problem is compounded because the drugs used may be treating conditions that in themselves can cause ED. Good examples are drugs for high blood pressure, depression and cholesterol lowering. Many recreational drugs are also associated with ED. Sometimes a change in the class of drug can be helpful, but this should be discussed with your doctor carefully because these drugs should not be stopped without medical advice.

Table 5.1: *Medications that can cause ED*

Cardiovascular drugs	Recreational drugs
Thiazide diuretics	Alcohol
Beta-blockers	Marijuana
Calcium antagonists	Amphetamines
Centrally acting agents such as:	Cocaine
- methyldopa	Anabolic steroids
- clonidine	Heroin
- reserpine	Testosterone
- ganglion blockers	**Endocrine drugs**
Digoxin	Anti-androgens
Lipid-lowering agents	Oestrogens
ACE inhibitors	LHRH analogues
Psychotropic drugs	Testosterone
Testosterone	**Others**
Anxiolytics and hypnotics	Cimetidine and ranitidine
Tricyclic antidepressants	Metoclopramide
Selective serotonin reuptake inhibitors	Carbamazepine

How to ensure your partner is taking their medication effectively and safely

VICTORIA

The leaflet enclosed with all tablets for ED tells you how to use them and lists all the possible contraindications, as well as the side effects your partner might experience. However, although the medication works just as the leaflet says, over 50% of men stop using the drug after the first prescription and 72% of men discontinue after one year.

It seems such a pity that, having taken the courage to visit the doctor, the packet of tablets is put in a drawer and not used again, especially as they really are so effective and safe. Over 70% of men have improved erections using these drugs and three out of four men prefer to use the higher dose.

I am writing about these drugs in the order in which they were licensed, not because one is better than the other. We are very lucky to have the choice and there is variation in how people respond. The main reason for discontinuation is that men are not using the tablets properly. Everyone is different and what works for one doesn't always work for another, so here are some ideas which may well help you both to have a positive response to the medication.

You need to remember that men are not used to taking tablets like women. After all, women are often taking the contraceptive pill for years and get used to the idea, but men don't. There has been much misinformation about the safety of drugs for ED in the popular press. I know lots of men who have been prescribed an oral drug for erection problems, and when they get home their partners say "Are you sure they are safe, perhaps you shouldn't take them after all? What happens if you have a heart attack? What happens if the children find them? What happens if your penis stays hard for ever? Well, of course, some partners may not want their partners to be taking a drug and have a great erection. You have no idea how many pills get flushed down the toilet and disappear. So you do need to talk about the consequences of taking a drug for ED. The drugs for ED have been thoroughly researched and are perfectly safe when used following the manufacturers' instructions.

Starting to have sex again after a break

If you have not had sex for many years and the vagina has not had anything inside it for a very long time, it will be quite a shock! So it is definitely time to talk to your partner, to find some lubricant and go to the doctor for a vaginal examination, just so you know that everything is healthy inside. I suggest that before you go to the doctor, lie in the bath and place your finger inside your vagina; you can tell when you touch the cervix because it feels a little like the end of your nose. Have a feel about and check that there is no discomfort; if all seems well, a rigid hard penis placed in the vagina will be fine, but a good lubricant is a must, especially the first time, and I don't mean just inside the vagina, but also placed all over the penis.

Now, I know that many of you will say, "but I am aroused and I feel wet, so why do we need a lubricant?" The answer is that both your brains have become used to experiencing a sexual problem, and there may be some underlying anxiety about history repeating itself. However, I have found that if my patients add a lubricant a few times, the different sensations and feelings confuse the brain, so the normal 'performance anxiety' does not log on so quickly, if at all.

Once you know your vagina is healthy, it is time to think about how to take the drugs. I know that by now you will have read all the information inside the packet and this is the time when we get worried – is the drug safe?

The doctor who prescribed the drug will know your partner's medical history and would not have prescribed the drug if they were worried about any potential problems. That is why it is so important not to buy any of these tablets from a friend or from a website, especially the first time, as these other sources are not aware of your personal health status. Most of all, nitrates are contraindicated. These are the drugs that are often given to patients to help relieve an angina attack.

When any drug is used for the first time it is natural to feel a little anxious. I believe it is important that men tell their partners they are using the drug – after all, nobody wants to be too surprised! If a partner lies about taking the drug, what else they may be lying about? So, best be honest.

Many men say to me "I am not going to tell my partner, I am going to surprise them!" Some of these couples have not had intercourse for 30 years. Well, it would be a surprise to wake up to a rigid penis next to you after all those years! There is a lovely story of a man in his 80s who thought he would surprise his new wife on her birthday. He decided to wake her up in the middle of the night, and place her hand on his hard penis. She screamed and said "Who are you?" "I am your loving husband," he replied. She screamed "If I had wanted a potent man I would have married one!"

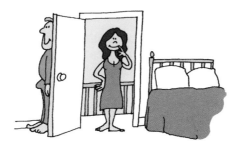

Remember, it is a myth that sex is spontaneous. Some of the best sex is when we talk about how intimate we want to be with one another; remember in those early days all those telephone calls, texts and loving notes you sent before you saw one another? After all, if we are planning to have friends around for dinner we plan what food we are going to give them, so why not plan our intimate time together; it is just as special, if not more so.

Treatment

Viagra (sildenafil)

Viagra is the blue pill and it comes in different strengths – 25, 50 and 100mgs. It is absorbed quickly and is a short-acting drug, in that it often clears through the body in about four to five hours. There has been some new research that tells us the drug lasts for longer, but you will not find out until you have started to use it. I would suggest that, for the first few tablets, you don't necessarily need to have sex, just try getting used to the sensations.

The doctor will have prescribed the dose that he thinks is the best for your partner to take. Some of my patients who are worried about side effects prefer to start on a lower dose and gradually increase it – it is up to you.

Whether your partner has been given 25, 50 or 100mgs, I suggest that, for the first time, he takes one tablet on his own. I would also suggest that he waits an hour to let the drug absorb into the system. Next he needs to place some lubricant on his penis and start to touch his penis for at least 20 minutes to see what sort of erection he gets. It does help to put a fantasy into your head at this point or at least find a good erotic magazine. You need to use all your senses for maximum effect. Now I know this may sound a little strange, asking your partner to pleasure himself, but the advantage is that he gets used to what happens when the drug works. He will also notice if he gets any side effects. These are, most commonly, a slightly red face and perhaps a bit of a headache. Some men get a slight blue haze to their vision but this doesn't last long and is not harmful.

The side effects will usually all disappear after he has taken the first four to eight tablets on different occasions. I would leave at least three days between tablets. The doctor will probably only have prescribed four tablets anyway, as the government guidelines are restricted to up to a pill a week on the NHS, although there is some flexibility on this issue. When starting treatment, more frequent dosing may be helpful.

The side effects are just the body getting used to the drug – this is the time to remember that if there is a slight headache, not to panic. Just take some mild painkillers. The side effects will pass more quickly if you are able to sit or lie down and relax after you have had sex.

As Clive Gingell, a respected urologist says: "There is only one thing better than the sleep of the just, and that is the sleep of the just after."

Please remember that these drugs are not an aphrodisiac; they do not work unless the penis is stimulated. You are not going to get an instant spontaneous erection watching Match of the Day or reading the newspaper.

You have no idea how many men come back to the clinic saying the drug has not worked. I ask if there was any direct foreplay to the penis and they look bewildered. They often reply, "I have never had to touch my penis before, so why now?" The answer is that the penis has not been working well and these tablets need sexual stimulation. So if you or your partner don't touch and stimulate the penis, it has been a complete waste of time and money.

Now, of course, some of you will want to try having intercourse on the first day, but I would still say keep to solo or mutual masturbation, and don't think about vaginal intercourse. It will help in the future because the first time you make love again you will be more confident about what to expect from taking the drug.

I like to think of an erection on a scale of hardness, ie one is soft and four is hard. You can imagine hardness using this scale:

- **Grade One:** Place your tongue inside your cheek – that's grade one
- **Grade Two:** Put your finger on the outside of your cheek – that's grade two
- **Grade Three:** Place your finger on the end of your nose – that's a grade three
- **Grade Four:** Place your finger on your forehead – that's a grade four

Grade 1: Marshmallow

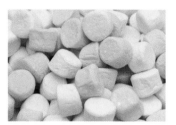

Grade2: Peeled banana

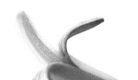

Grade 3: Unpeeled banana

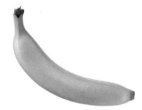

Grade 4: Cucumber

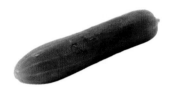

Your partner's erection was probably about a grade one, two or three before and what you are both aiming for is a grade four.

So, if he has taken the first tablet and both of you don't think the penis is hard enough, and there have been no side effects you could increase the dose. Remember, 100mgs is the highest dose and it is not wise to increase above 100mgs. If the first dose was 25mgs I would increase it to 50mgs. If the dosage was 50mgs, I would stay at that dose one more time and increase the foreplay.

The problem with going straight to the 100mgs is that you are likely to get more side effects at this early stage of taking the drug, and you may not need the higher dose anyway. After your partner has taken about four doses of the drugs at separate times you will work out which is the best dosage for you both. What you do need to remember with Viagra, is that if you have a very heavy meal and lots of alcohol, the drug will take longer to work, so think about what you have eaten during the day, as this will make a difference. Also, I would suggest that in the early stages you don't take the drug and think of having sexual activity very late at night after a long day at work. You will just to be too tired to concentrate on that loving touch. Daylight hours are best, with at least half an hour of foreplay, including direct touch to the penis. However, this is completely a matter for each couple to decide; there is no 'right' or 'wrong'.

If your partner has been having erection difficulties for a long while, it is likely that it will take a little longer to find the best dose, so don't rush things. I would say it is best not to move onto another drug until you have tried at least four to six separate tablets of the same dosage. Additionally, if the side effects are intolerable, lower the dose; the side effects nearly always reduce over time and eventually go away, so just persevere – you will soon see the benefits.

Levitra (vardenafil)

Levitra is a peachy coloured pill, and comes in three different doses – 5, 10 and 20mgs. It is absorbed into the body quickly, but this does not mean that you should have less foreplay or genital stimulation. You don't need to be too worried about what you have eaten before, as it absorbs well unless you have a high fat meal. The side effects are a possible headache, along with flushing and dyspepsia. These will pass as your body gets used to the drug.

It is short acting and clears from the body in about five hours and many people say it is very similar to Viagra. That would be like saying that every Hoover is the same. However, Levitra and Viagra are absorbed quickly, so sex can be planned and prepared for in a short time. Some patients report that the effect of one tablet lasts at least two to three days!

You will need to follow the same instructions as for Viagra above to make sure that you get the best results.

Cialis (tadalafil)

Cialis comes in two doses – 10 and 20mgs and is a yellow tablet. It is slightly different from Viagra and Levitra, in that it has a longer half life, ie it stays in the bloodstream longer, giving you the potential advantage of being effective for 24 – 36 hours.

This is how I suggest that you take the first four to eight tablets. Make sure you and your partner plan when to take the drug; I would suggest that your partner takes the drug twice a week at the 10mgs dose, for example on a Tuesday and a Friday. Do this for least two weeks. Your partner may notice that his erections in the morning will be harder. If he is not experiencing any side effects and there is only a slight change to the morning erections, in other words they are only a little harder, increase the dose to 10mgs on a Tuesday and 20mgs on the Friday. During this time I would suggest that he masturbates solo on occasions to determine the effect.

Remember, when you are starting to use a drug, you are just trying to find out what suits you both – you cannot fail and you will be a lot wiser.

Cialis has only a few side effects, like flushing and headaches, but it can give you some muscle ache in the back. If this happens, either lower the dose for a while and take some painkillers if necessary. Remember – the side effects nearly always go away, so don't panic.

Men who have not been experiencing early morning erections often report a real "hard on" in the early hours after using these drugs. This is not because you are lying next to them, or they are fantasising, or that they have a full bladder. It is because they are experiencing something which we call REM sleep. This type of sleep relaxes the nerve pathways so much that it gives the genitals more blood flow and, no, he doesn't have to use that erection to have sex with you. Let it just go down, and be pleased to know that the penis is showing signs of being healthy again.

Cialis needs just as much touch to the genitals and foreplay to work as the other drugs, but as it lasts longer in the bloodstream, giving you more spontaneity, less planning before sex and an opportunity to have sex without taking a pill just before the event. On the other hand, many men prefer to take a short acting drug that is quickly absorbed and when they feel the first flush of blood to the skin they know they are ready for sex.

We often find that once a man and his partner have tried all of the ED medication, they can make a decision as to which of the drugs suits best. Some prefer a short-acting tablet during the week like Viagra or Levitra and use Cialis at the weekend. Ultimately the choice is yours.

Intracavernosal injection therapy

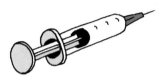

After an injection with alprostadil, you can expect to obtain an erection within 5-20 minutes and it may last for approximately 30 minutes. It will occur whether or not sexual stimulation is present, although subsequent sexual stimulation will enhance the effects.

The initial injection should be given by a medical professional demonstrating the sterile technique and monitoring the response to the injected agent. It is helpful also for the partner to be present, especially as it is often the partner who will carry out the injection, helping to make it seem an acceptable part of a normal lovemaking act.

The erection should be monitored for rigidity and duration, and if this is adequate, then the injections can be prescribed for self administration. Alprostadil is usually started as a dose of 1.25µg in patients with a normal blood supply to the penis and 2.5µg for older patients or those who are known to have vascular disease. Doses can be prescribed up to 20µg.

After retracting the foreskin, hold the penis firmly in the non-dominant hand and inject the drug slowly into the side of the shaft of the penis with the syringe perpendicular to the skin, taking care not to hit any of the large subcutaneous veins which are usually visible. Once the needle is removed, firm pressure is applied to the injection site and the drug is massaged gently throughout the shaft of the penis for approximately 30 seconds. Sometimes, men find it helpful to walk around the room to increase the blood flow.

Despite the effectiveness of this type of treatment, there has always been a very high dropout rate, which is usually due to discomfort from the injection, lack of spontaneity and inadequate erectile function. With regard to pain, it is very important to inject the substance very slowly. Be warned that injection induced erections often do not subside immediately after ejaculation and may persist for an hour or two in some cases. However, if an erection lasts for more than four hours, you must seek immediate medical attention. Delayed treatment of a prolonged erection can result in damage to the corpus cavernosum and permanent or complete loss of erectile function.

There are certain people who cannot use injection therapy, such as patients who have leukaemia, sickle cell disease and significant coagulation (blood clotting) problems, as well as men using oral anticoagulants for heart disease.

Transurethral drug application (MUSE)

Figure 5.1: *Transurethral application of alprostadil*

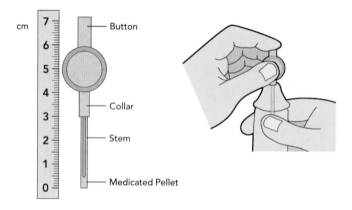

Intraurethral delivery of alprostadil (Medicated Urethral System for Erection, MUSE) provides a less invasive alternative to intracavernosal injection. It is important to pass urine first because a small amount of urine in the urethra helps the pellet to dissolve. A small (1.4mm) pellet is inserted with the aid of an applicator into the urethra 15 minutes before intercourse is planned. The drug quickly dissolves after insertion and gets absorbed into the corpora cavernosum. It should lead to an erection which lasts for 30-60 minutes.

The pellets are available in concentrations of 125, 250, 500 and 1000μg of PGE1. The dose used is 50 times higher than the intracavernosal injection because a significant amount of the drug will enter the general circulation and never reach the corpora cavernosum. Efficacy can be increased by massage and using a constriction band at the base of the penis, which is applied prior to the administration of the pellet.

MUSE can be used up to twice daily. The main side effects are discomfort and tenderness within the penis. Sometimes it may cause vaginal discomfort and itching in the female partner. MUSE is not recommended for use with pregnant partners. It is also a good idea to use a condom if you are having oral sex, because if the pellet has not been completely absorbed it could be "sucked" up by your partner!

Vacuum constriction devices

Figure 5.2: Use of a vacuum constriction device

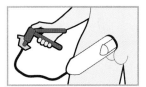 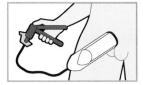

Medical literature suggests that vacuum pumps were first used to enhance penile function as early as the late 1800s. In 1917 the vacuum constriction device was patented by Dr Otto Lederer. Acceptance of this management approach has increased with the development of a modern vacuum constriction device. There are currently many companies that manufacture these devices and there is an excellent choice. The device is composed of three main parts, a cylinder with an open end to which the penis is inserted, a vacuum pump that is operated either by hand or battery, and a constriction ring.

The penis is placed into the cylinder and the cylinder is pumped to produce a vacuum. The vacuum should be applied for approximately six minutes. Many manufacturers recommend pumping for one to two minutes, releasing pressure and then resuming pumping for three to four minutes. Once an erection is produced, the constriction ring is slipped off the cylinder onto the base of the penis, to maintain the erection. The ring should not be worn for more than 30 minutes at a time. The device should be used with caution in men with bleeding or clotting disorders as they run the risk of significant bruising, particularly at the site of the constriction ring.

Please buy a pump from a reputable manufacturer and not a sex shop. Using a pump regularly improves the natural response. The penis is sometimes a little cold after using the pump, especially at the start of treatment. Some of my patients use those small face cloths that you are given in Chinese restaurants; they wrap it around the penis just before intercourse. If a man is particularly hairy in the pubic region he may want to trim the hairs and use plenty of lubricant to gain better suction.

The biggest reason for dropout is that men complain that using a device can be cumbersome and interrupts sexual relations. However, these devices will produce an erection in 92% of patients, regardless of the underlying cause of ED.

Surgical treatment for ED

Surgery may be considered in the case of certain conditions, or if all other treatment options have failed, are unacceptable or are contraindicated. Penile prostheses have a high success rate and do provide a one off solution. However, they do have a higher incidence of complications than the other treatments. Because they are mechanical devices, they can eventually malfunction and may require replacement at a later date. Also, there is the risk of infection and many men find that the size of the penis decreases. Lastly, they are very expensive.

TOP TIPS

on talking to your partner ...

- Read the information you have been given together
- Underline anything that you don't understand and see if one of you has the answers; if not speak to your doctor
- Talk about how you might increase foreplay
- Discuss how you are going to make sure you make love when you are not too tired, or after a heavy night
- Go shopping for some lingerie and a lubricant
- Erections are good for erections
- Don't have a high fat meal before taking viagra or levitra
- If the tablets don't work, don't give up, see your doctor to discuss
- Avoid taking too much alcohol
- Allow the drugs time to work
- Don't give up after one or two tablets
- The longer erections have been absent, the more tablets will be required over a longer time to get a response

Urological problems

Let me tell you a story

VICTORIA

When I was a chorister about aged 11, I was a quiet and shy girl; I was always terribly embarrassed when it came to talking about anything personal. One day, as I was walking to church, I knew I should have gone to the toilet before I left home. When I got to the church, I couldn't bring myself to "pee" in the churchyard behind a grave. In those days I had no idea were the nearest toilet was, so I put on my gown and hat and walked down the aisle singing. I was just about OK, until I got to the prayer time, when I was kneeling down on the cushion, and I thought to myself if I just let a little urine out I will manage to get through the service, but of course, once the flow started it never stopped and before long there was steam rising and I was kneeling in a large puddle. You can imagine my horror as within 10 minutes I would have to walk down the aisle; goodness knows how I managed. But I do remember wrapping my blue gown around me and running.

There must have been someone very kind in the choir, because the next time I went to church my gown was clean and fresh. No one ever mentioned the mishap, but I learnt a very good lesson, if you want to go, don't hold on. It is less embarrassing talking and asking where to go to find a toilet rather than risk a mishap!

Urine and bowel problems do affect our sex lives. First of all, when we experience a pain or symptoms related to that part of our anatomy, we often feel that that area is 'sick' and when it is touched it reminds us of the symptoms we are worrying about.

There is nothing worse than to start being intimate with one another and then find that you want to empty your bladder. You worry that you might lose control and become incontinent during sex. This embarrassment leads to couples refusing any further intimacy. So do empty your bladder and don't be anxious about sharing your worries with your loved one, especially if you have been suffering from urinary problems.

MIKE

Lower urinary tract symptoms

These include frequency of passing urine, urgency to pass urine, urge incontinence, night time urination, difficulty passing urine, ie poor stream, straining, stopping and starting, and pain on passing urine. Pain is an important symptom and should be reported to your GP.

There is a known association between lower urinary tract symptoms (LUTS) and ED, and both should be discussed with your GP. Aging of the bladder causes a condition known as overactive bladder and typical symptoms include frequency, urgency and night time urination. These symptoms can be improved with a bladder retraining programme. (See Appendix III on page 107)

LUTS can be caused by enlargement of the prostate, which is a gland that encircles the neck of the bladder. The prostate is normally the size of a chestnut but can increase to the size of a mandarin in older men. As it increases in size it causes obstruction to the flow of urine as it comes out of the bladder, which in turn causes symptoms of overactive bladder. There are medications that will shrink the prostate, but these do have some sexual side effects in terms of reduced libido (Dutasteride and Finasteride). Other drugs used to treat LUTS are alpha-blockers, which relax the neck of the bladder (Tamsulosin).

TOP TIP

■ ED and urinary symptoms often occur together. If you are having problems with urinary symptoms or urinary control and have ED, don't ignore it – talk to your doctor.

CASE STUDY 5

Tom was 62 years old and had been experiencing urinary problems, getting up in the night, dribbling and not emptying his bladder properly. He went to the hospital and underwent some tests and was examined for prostate problems.

He had decided to sleep separately because he had not wanted to disturb his wife's sleep. She was working and also experiencing menopausal night sweats, so it was a difficult time for them both.

When I saw them in clinic, they also admitted to very little foreplay, because every time Tom was touched on the penis it reminded him and his wife of his symptoms. They had often had oral sex but this had also been put on the back burner. So, in fact, the bladder problems not only caused a high level of anxiety but also stopped this couple from being intimate.

It was suggested that Tom massaged urine out of his bladder. Urine tends to collect in the down pipe, and if a man massages the base of the penis behind the testicles forwards, he can express any urine that has collected. Also pelvic floor muscles get weaker as one gets older, so it is a good idea to improve the pelvic muscle tone by doing regular pelvic floor exercises.

Prostate gland

The prostate gland is part of the male genitourinary system. It is a small organ that lies just below the bladder. It surrounds the urethra, the tube that carries urine from the bladder out of the body through the penis. The prostate gland produces most of the fluid in the semen. In the past, doctors and patients alike have been led to believe that both male sexual problems and urinary problems are just an inevitable consequence of aging. This misconception, coupled with a man's natural reluctance to discuss any embarrassing problems, has led to many couples believing that nothing can be done. Nowadays, however, knowledge of male sexual function and the workings of the prostate gland and bladder have increased considerably and, as a result, there are many good treatments available for the majority of men.

Figure 6.1: Diagram showing location of prostate gland

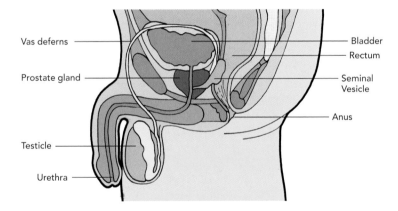

There is no doubt that both male sexual dysfunction and prostate disease increase with age and approximately half of all men aged 40-70 years admit to some level of erection problems and bothersome urinary symptoms. Prostate cancer is rare before the age of 40 and more than 80% of cases are diagnosed in men over the age of 65. From birth to young adulthood, the prostate gland grows from the size of a pea to about the size of a walnut. Most men experience a second period of prostate growth after the age of 40.

There are primarily three conditions that affect the prostate gland:

1. Benign prostatic hyperplasia (BPH)

This is enlargement of the prostate and is the most common condition to affect the prostate. It does eventually cause problems because it obstructs the flow of urine out of the bladder. The back pressure effect causes consequent bladder problems, symptoms of which include frequency in passing urine, getting up at night to pass urine, reduced urinary stream and often hesitancy in starting to urinate. There are medical treatments available for this condition, which are very effective.

Treatment for BPH

A course of tablets are first line therapy. TURP is a common operation for the treatment of BPH, which involves part of the prostate that is blocking the urethra (the tube that carries urine from the bladder to the exterior), being removed via an instrument inserted down the urethra through the penis. This sounds uncomfortable but most men recover very quickly from this surgical procedure.

Sexual side effects associated with TURP can include semen that flows backwards into the bladder during ejaculation, known as retrograde ejaculation and sometimes problems with erection (ED). Retrograde ejaculation is when a man experiences the sensation of ejaculation but no fluid emerges. What has happened is that the semen passes into the bladder and then out of the body in the urine instead of out the body through the penis in orgasm. It does not normally cause ED and does not affect the sensation of orgasm. It does no harm but it does reduce fertility and the chances of fathering a child. Laser treatment is another method of performing surgery. With laser treatment, bleeding is less common and the technique is probably less likely than TURP to affect ejaculation.

Table 6.1: BPH treatments linked to sexual problems[6]

Treatment	Potential sexual side effects
Tablets – alpha blockers	Retrograde ejaculation, but the effect is reversible
Tablets – 5-alpha reductase inhibitors	Erection problems, loss of libido and reduction in ejaculate volume
Surgery – Transurethral Resection of the Prostate (TURP)	Retrograde ejaculation, rarely erection problems
Surgery – Transurethral Incision of the Prostate (TUIP)	Much lower risk of retrograde ejaculation than with TURP
Surgery – Open prostatectomy	Similar risk of retrograde ejaculation as TURP, possibility of erection problems
Surgery – Laser prostatectomy	Lower risk of retrograde ejaculation than with TURP

2. Prostate cancer

This is the most common form of cancer to affect men and there will be approximately 30,000 men in the UK diagnosed with it this year. The condition is normally diagnosed by means of a blood test, the PSA test, or by a digital rectal examination (DRE), which allows the doctor to feel the size of the prostate gland to determine whether there are any small lumps within it. There are some very effective treatments for prostate cancer, but early detection is important.

Treatment for prostate cancer
Treatment for prostate cancer is linked to sexual problems

Table 6.2: *Prostate cancer treatments linked to sexual problems*[6]

Treatment	Potential sexual side effects
Hormone treatments	Erection problems, decreased libido, side effects can be reversed on stopping therapy
Surgery – Radical prostatectomy	No ejaculate, erection problems
Radiotherapy	Erection problems + reduced ejaculate volume
Surgery – Orchidectomy (surgical removal of the testes)	Loss of libido, fertility and ability to attain an erection. Effects are irreversible

Some of the treatments for prostate diseases can cause sexual problems and Table 6.2 above provides information about this.

3. Prostatitis

Prostatitis is an inflammatory disease of the prostate, which is less common than BPH or prostate cancer and generally affects younger men. Prostatitis can cause pain and discomfort around the anus, scrotum and the area in between.

Prostatitis can be caused by both viruses and bacteria. The bacterial causes of prostatitis are commonly treated with antibiotics, which do not generally cause significant sexual side effects. However, having experienced discomfort in the groin caused by prostatitis can lead to ED and lack of interest in sex, especially when there is chronic pelvic pain.

Treatment for prostatitis

Unfortunately, there are no universally effective treatments for chronic prostatitis. The doctor may prescribe antibiotics, anti-inflammatory tablets, anti-neuralgic tablets and sometimes an alpha-blocker tablet which is commonly used for BPH.

We do know that at times of illness, we have to place our energy into coping with our health problems and although intercourse and arousal may not be our priority, in times of crisis, intimacy and physical closeness reminds us that we are supported and loved.

CASE STUDY 6

Radical Prostatectomy

30,000 men will be diagnosed with prostate cancer and this year Ben was one of them. He is only 56 and had a loving wife. They made love at least once or twice per week and a diagnosis of prostate cancer at a routine screening visit for general health came as a bolt out of the blue. The tumour was aggressive and a radical prostatectomy operation was performed as a matter of urgency. No-one had time or perhaps thought it was important to discuss the sexual implications of this surgery, which left him with a total inability to get an erection.

It took the couple 18 months to finally get around to presenting with the problem. Because there had been no erections for such a long time, treatment was not, however, totally successful. Erections are good for erections. The night time and spontaneous erections that occur in normal healthy men basically help to keep the penis healthy.

We learnt a lot from this couple and many specialist units around the world now recommend the early institution of a rehabilitation programme after radical prostatectomy.

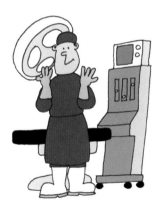

Restoring erections and keeping the penis healthy after radical prostatectomy

There is no doubt that restoring erections at an early stage may improve the speed of recovery of normal erections in men who have had a radical prostatectomy. The important nerves and blood vessels to the penis run very close to the prostate gland, and can often get damaged, bruised or occasionally even cut during surgery. Of course, the surgeon's main aim is to remove all the cancer but they will do their very best to preserve the nerves and blood vessels to the penis whenever possible.

Many men will experience a prolonged absence of erections after surgery and unfortunately during this period of time there is some loss of muscle fibres within the penile erectile tissue (the corpora cavernosum). Many specialists will now offer men oral therapy initially with tablets such as sildenafil (Viagra), vardenafil (Levitra) and tadalafil (Cialis). These tablets should be taken regularly from an early stage, aiming to keep the penis healthy while waiting for recovery, which may take up to two years. Injections and vacuum devices are also advised in some specialised centres.

After the operation

You should attempt to get an erection, either with self stimulation or with stimulation by your partner, as soon as you feel motivated to do so after removal of your catheter and try this at least every other day. This is an important part of the rehabilitation programme. If you are not able to get an erection without medication, you should try taking one of the tablets that are prescribable under the NHS, to assist the process. If you have heart disease or are taking other medications, your doctor will first need to check that these drugs are appropriate for you. Do not buy them over the internet.

If you wish, you can start taking these medications as soon as your catheter has been removed, but do not leave it longer than six weeks after your operation to start the programme. You should take the tablet one to two hours before trying to get an erection and you should do this (at least) every other day. But remember, the pills will not work without stimulation, although with regular dosing night time erections may start to return.

A further important measure is to start to use a vacuum erection device, and you can do this as soon as the discomfort from the operation has worn off. The vacuum device may cause some pain if it is used too early due to pressure at the base of the penis. Most men are quite comfortable by one month or so after the surgery. Try and remember to use the vacuum device twice per day and without the constriction ring, unless you plan to attempt intercourse. The vacuum device will allow you to fill the penis with blood and you should maintain this for a few minutes before releasing the pressure.

If these measures fail, then there are alternatives, which include injection therapy (Caverject) or a tablet which is placed in the urethra, known as transurethral therapy (MUSE). We normally recommend trying the tablets and the vacuum device first, because although 70% of men will get a good erection with the injection therapy, it can occasionally cause pain and discomfort and sometimes fibrosis of the penis, when the tissues within the corpora cavernosum thicken up and become lumpy.

The transurethral therapy (when a tiny pellet is passed into the urethra of the penis with a device [MUSE]) is not as effective as the injections, but works in 40-50% of men. It can cause some discomfort in the penis and occasionally, like the injections, a prolonged erection known as priapism. After these therapies, if you have an erection that lasts more than four hours, you must seek medical attention.

Remember that the nerves will take a long time to recover and the aim of the rehabilitation programme is to keep the penis healthy while waiting for the recovery to occur, so don't give up!

TOP TIPS

on urology ...

- LUTS are very common for men and women over 50
- Bladder retraining and pelvic floor exercises are very effective
- Not all LUTS are due to prostate disease
- All bleeding should be reported to your doctor
- Men should not get urinary infections, there is usually a cause
- Women get fewer infections if they pass urine after sexual intercourse or if they use topical HRT
- After prostate operations start penile rehabilitation early
- Empty bladder before sex
- But don't get dehydrated!

CHAPTER 7

Testosterone deficiency – men have hormones, too!

MIKE

Testosterone deficiency is a rare cause of ED. If it is suspected, then blood should be taken at 9am to confirm the diagnosis and repeated on a further one or two occasions. Testosterone therapy with injections, patches or gels is only indicated in men whose loss of libido or ED is due to a proven lack of testosterone. Failure to respond to the normal drugs for treating ED may also indicate testosterone deficiency and taking additional testosterone in this situation can then make the drugs effective.

Because lack of testosterone can cause subtle symptoms, some doctors use questionnaires. Questionnaires may help to reduce feelings of embarrassment that arise when talking about sexual problems. The ADAM questionnaire is one way to establish whether a man's low testosterone level may account for his erection problems. The questionnaire includes 10 questions that have a yes or no answer (see page 68). A positive response to questions 1 or 7, or any other three questions, suggests the need to have an early morning (9am) testosterone blood test.

With increasing age, there is a fall in testosterone levels in most men and this coincides with many other hormone changes that take place simultaneously. Additionally, with increasing age, there are a number of changes that occur in sexual performance. Often the libido will be decreased, penile sensitivity is diminished and it takes longer for full erection to be achieved.

In older men the higher centres of the brain are less reactive to psychogenic stimuli such as fantasising or visual stimuli, so the erections become more dependent on manual stimulation. Increased interaction between the couple, especially in terms of foreplay, is needed to achieve a satisfactory erection. There is a decrease in the frequency, duration and rigidity of nocturnal erections and an increase in the refractory period (the time from ejaculation to the next erection). This interval may range from 30 minutes in a young man, to several days in an 80 year old enthusiast! Many older men fail to recognise that they need longer to become aroused; this delay could lead to increased performance related anxiety, which in turn could lead to a vicious circle, resulting in a complete loss of erectile function.

The ADAM questionnaire

1. Do you have decreasing libido?
2. Do you have lack of energy?
3. Do you have a decrease in strength or endurance?
4. Have you lost height?
5. Have you decreased enjoyment of life?
6. Are you sad or grumpy?
7. Are your erections less strong?
8. Is it difficult to maintain your erection?
9. Are you falling asleep after dinner?
10. Has your work performance deteriorated recently?

CASE STUDY 7

Robert was 52, in a very happy relationship but complained of constantly feeling tired and he could not be bothered to initiate sexual activity. His erections had also been unpredictable and when he ejaculated he felt as if some of the pleasure had diminished.

His girlfriend was worried, not so much about this erections, but the fact that he had not initiated sex seemed unusual, especially as they were so much in love.

This is when it is so important to talk to a specialist. On the surface it seems that at 52, Robert was just tired from work and it could be said that as the relationship was a few years old, sex would not be so regular. Some men, when they experience these symptoms go onto internet sites and complete questionnaires and then either buy testosterone treatment on the web or spend an enormous amount of money at expensive private clinics in London. (continued on next page)

This is not necessary and can be dangerous. First of all, if you take testosterone when your hormone levels are normal, you create a tremendous risk of shutting down the whole hormonal feedback system, and it may never recover; there are serious long term health consequences to using testosterone unsupervised. Secondly, some clinics outside the NHS prescribe testosterone without necessarily following all the appropriate guidelines and tests associated with treatment.

If anyone has concerns as to whether their testosterone levels are low, the first point of call is your local doctor to explain your symptoms and worries, and to ask for your hormone levels to be measured. It is still best to have a 9am check; you do not need to fast but the levels do change throughout the day and therefore a 9am test gives you the best levels. Testosterone levels can be low for a number of reasons, and I cannot stress enough how important it is to see an appropriate specialist.

Robert was found to have a high level of prolactin which lowers testosterone. The tests showed a small tumour, which was benign, and was treated accordingly. He was then placed on testosterone treatment, which made a considerable difference to his sex life and their relationship.

TOP TIPS

- If you have a significant score on the ADAM questionnaire, discuss the matter with your doctor and a testosterone blood test may be helpful.

- One abnormal testosterone test is not reliable and does need to be repeated to confirm the result.

- There is a wide range of normal testosterone levels; what might be low for one man may be normal for another.

- A trial of treatment can sometimes be helpful.

- If you are not getting a good response to the tablets prescribed for ED, then it is worth discussing the possibility of a low testosterone with your doctor.

- Testosterone treatment can turn a non-responder into a responder if they are truly testosterone deficient.

- Many of the changes that occur in erectile function in older men are a normal part of aging and not related to a low testosterone.

- The best way to stay fit for sex in older age is to keep your weight down, be moderate with alcohol, be a non-smoker, take plenty of exercise and eat a healthy, balanced diet.

CHAPTER 8

Menopause

VICTORIA

One of the most common reasons why women in the menopausal years shy away from sexual activity is because they have bladder problems. There are some studies that show that 50% of women with urge incontinence, sometimes described as an overactive bladder, are likely to be incontinent at orgasm and many women avoid becoming too sexually aroused and stop short of being orgasmic, in case they are incontinent.

In the USA there is more money spent on adult incontinence pads than children's nappies. Many women, rather than risk leaking or having to suddenly break off from sexual activity, often just give up sex; the sad thing is that there are a variety of treatments available if only we ask.

Many of my patients give up foreplay, especially oral sex, but they forget to tell their partners, often just pushing them away and saying no. The partner then tends to enter the vagina with a slightly softer penis, and everything is over in seconds: unsatisfactory sex and, of course, if sex is not pleasurable, why go back for more?

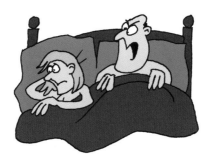

In the menopausal years our faces lose their lustre and become wrinkly and vaginas become shiny and smooth – just the opposite of what we need for pain free sex! This is called atrophic vaginitis and affects 10% – 40% of post menopausal women. It can lead to:

- Pain on intercourse
- Reduced vaginal lubrication
- Performance anxiety
- Loss of sexual desire to initiate sex
- Relationship distress and lack of intimacy
- Avoidance of sexual relationships

Unfortunately, doctors don't always ask about the health of our vagina; this is partly because the "ticket" we have used in the past when we discuss HRT has gone. So many women are now worried about the side effects of HRT, as well as the embarrassment of undergoing a vaginal examination and the fear of what else the doctor might find, that they are walking around unaware that their vaginas have less oestrogen, which means that the cushioning effect we have when a penis enters us has been reduced. Hence, we get that pain and soreness and even urinary problems. Pain is the greatest inhibitor of sexual activity which is why we need to get treatment for these symptoms.

When a man enters you and you experience discomfort, you may think to yourself: "This is not much fun, let's not to do it again." So it's separate bedtimes and bedrooms as quickly as possible.

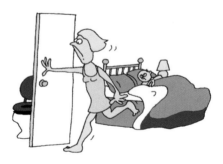

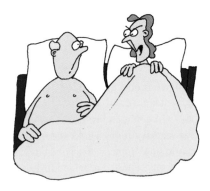

Imagine an upholstered chair which is comfortable to sit on, and then imagine yourself sitting on a hard chair and the discomfort associated with that. That is what happens to your vagina. It also loses its elasticity.

Most women, I believe, want to be given the information about HRT. They can then make an informed decision about possible treatment. Certainly, if your quality of life has deteriorated because of sleepless nights, hot sweats and mood changes, HRT can be the answer. However, there is always the choice of using a special hormonal cream, which will provide you with a nice spongy soft, plumped up vagina, and then there will be no pain and no urinary symptoms. Now that so many men are taking treatments to improve their erections, we women must look after our vaginas – if not, only one of you will have healthy genitals.

Another problem in the menopause is that our senses seem to alter. That means that the touch and smells we have enjoyed before become irritating and often not very arousing. I have known women who for years have really enjoyed their face being touched or their arm stroked, and then for some reason, the touch their partner gives them is annoying and not a 'turn on'. The main problem is that we forget to tell our partners about this change and they go on, for years sometimes, still touching the same place, wondering why it is no longer enjoyable.

Please tell them it is not them you are criticising, it is their actions that you want them to change. Just because a partner has been with you for years, it does not mean he can or should be able to read your mind.

MIKE

Vaginal atrophy in the menopause from a male doctor's point of view

Menopausal symptoms of hot flushes, night sweats and mood changes are well known and can be effectively treated with hormone replacement therapy (HRT). A common problem in the menopause which can cause sexual difficulties is vaginal atrophy. Under the influence of oestrogen, the vaginal lining is thick, elastic, and supple, with a good blood supply which allows fluid from the capillaries in the vagina to provide lubrication and moisture. In addition to this, mucous production from the glands adds to lubrication. Lactic acid produced in the vagina by healthy bacteria keeps the vagina acid, which provides resistance against infection.

Reduced oestrogen, associated with the menopause, leads to reduced blood supply and thereby less moisture and reduced mucous production. The lining of the vagina becomes dry, thin and fragile with reduced elasticity. There is less colonisation by the important lactobacilli, which leads to less lactic acid production and increased susceptibility to infection. Unfortunately, these changes can be made worse by smoking and they are also more common in women who have not given birth vaginally.

Vaginal atrophy can occur before the menopause, when the oestrogen levels are low. The diagnosis is made from the symptoms and by an examination. An examination will reveal the vulva to lack plumpness, the labia minora to be small, the vagina to appear thin, pale and dry and sometimes little blood spots known as petechiae may be present. Some specialists measure the acidity of the vagina to help make the diagnosis.

Reduced lubrication on sexual arousal is often one of the first symptoms of vaginal atrophy. Many women complain of vaginal dryness, which can lead to reduced sensation and discomfort during intercourse. Any discomfort or pain naturally leads to decreased interest in, and decreased frequency of, intercourse, which in turn leads to further decreases in vaginal lubrication. In addition, thinning of the vaginal and vulval skin causes irritation and discomfort, even to a gentle touch. In some women the lining of the vagina may be so fragile that bleeding can occur after intercourse. Any bleeding after the menopause should be appropriately investigated and not be assumed to be due to age related changes.

Urinary symptoms can also be related to a lack of oestrogen; these include pain on passing urine, frequency, urgency and urge incontinence, together with night time passing of urine. There are safe and effective treatments for vaginal atrophy which come in the form of topical creams to rub into the skin or pessaries to insert into the vagina. Replens is a non-hormonal vaginal remoisturiser and can be of some help. However, it will not reverse all the local changes produced by the lack of oestrogen.

The treatments, vaginal creams, tablets or pessaries, are typically a single dose used each night for a fortnight then one dose twice per week. Some women will need higher doses for longer to achieve good symptom relief. There is some evidence that a maintenance dose twice weekly is more effective than once weekly.

TOP TIPS

- Menopause and vaginal problems are very common
- Good treatment is available that really makes a difference
- Try facing side to side
- Man on top, but not with the woman on her tummy
- Plenty of lubrication
- Plenty of foreplay – don't rush it
- Put a little bit in and then see how comfortable you are
- "Brace yourself, Sheila" is not good enough!
- A shiny smooth vagina is a sign of lack of oestrogen

CASE STUDY 8

VICTORIA

A couple came to see me many years ago, and I remember the lady's face was beautiful and she looked a lot like Julie Andrews; I always wanted to be a nun, so I remember her very clearly. Goodness knows how I changed direction to become a sex therapist!

This lady and her husband had been married for 30 years, and they had stopped being intimate. I asked him on his own what they always did as foreplay, and what turned them on. "I always kiss my wife goodnight and that kiss would lead to more touching and then intercourse." I asked, "Why are you not kissing anymore?" He replied, "Well, every night she puts this seaweed cream on her face, and it smells dreadful. I would have to hold my breath to kiss her, which is not possible." I asked, "Have you told her?" He replied, "No, my wife is very worried about looking older and I don't want to worry her." I asked him to tell her about the cream, and he agreed. Her reply was, "I hate the smell too, but I didn't want you to think that I didn't care about my complexion, and so I have been using it for you".

From that day, the cream was thrown away, they started kissing again, and intimacy returned. Simple, but a good lesson for us all – we must communicate!

CHAPTER 9

Are you in the right position?

VICTORIA

Variety – "the spice of life"

We know that the more creative and the greater sexual repertoire we have, the greater the chance of maintaining a good sex life. If I served you up the same meal, at the same time of day, in the same chair, at the same table, you would soon get bored and uninterested. We need to remember that sexual activity is much the same; we need variety, that thrill of trying something new together. It is this that keeps us as interested in sex as it does in eating.

Unfortunately, some couples get used to having sex at a particular time of day, with the lights off, three minutes of foreplay and then intercourse. When we go through the different stages of our life, we often have to adapt to family and work circumstances. It is not uncommon, for instance, for a newly married couple to prioritise their love making, because it is new and exciting, then children come along, and although the couple would like to have regular sexual activity, the woman may think, "I had better get this over quickly in case the children wake up", or, when the children are older they think "I had better be careful not to make too much noise in case they know what we are up to".

Parents often feel that it would be so embarrassing if their children were aware that they are having sex. We respond to this by having quick sex, and although a 'quickie' can be fun in the right circumstances, it is so easy to get into a bad habit and forget about the intimacy of sex, having time to cuddle and talk and explore one another's bodies rather than just aiming for orgasm.

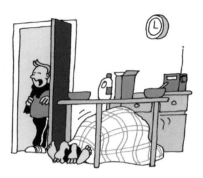

The main problem with having such a small repertoire of sexual activity and not trying out different ways of pleasuring one another, or different sexual positions, is this: when we get older and our bodies are suffering from arthritis, back pain, or we have had recent surgery such as a hip replacement or major heart surgery, we will often have to change or alter our sexual positions, so that we don't feel pain or get cramp, or to avoid the worry that we might damage ourselves in some way.

If we have never talked about different kinds of intimate contact and have not even talked about our sex lives, then if we get ill it is so much more difficult to change. I think this is partly because when a partner is ill, one of the couple becomes a carer for a while, and this alters the dynamic in the relationship. Carers are not supposed to ask for their needs to be met and so intimacy is often put to one side. Years later, couples say, "It all started when my wife had a hip replacement and started sleeping downstairs", or "When my husband had prostate problems, I didn't want to trouble him. Now that he is better I would love to have him back in bed with me, but we have got used to this new bedtime routine".

CASE STUDY 9

Mary and John had been married eight years and had two children aged five and three. Prior to the children, they enjoyed making love on Sunday afternoons. This was their special time, which they had prioritised just for them. During the week they both worked and had found that at weekends they were less tired and distracted. No problem until, of course, the children arrived and Sunday afternoons started to be filled with family activities.

Almost without them being aware, their Sunday afternoon intimacy disappeared. Neither of them had been used to having sex in the week and so, months passed without them having sex. When John had suggested they went to bed early, Mary had felt irritated as there was always so much to do around the house and, having looked after the needs of the children all day, she was frustrated that her husband seemed to want her to fulfil his sexual needs.

They attended the clinic worried that they had not been intimate for a long time, and both felt that their closeness as a couple had deteriorated and resentments had built up over time, which they could not resolve on their own.

This couple agreed that on one evening a week for 10 minutes, they would talk about their relationship, what worked well and what needed to change. They would then prioritise one concern and discuss how they could help one another cope with the problem better. This is a special way of coping with problems, as blame never produces a good outcome. We are often attracted to a person because they have qualities that we lack and that we admire in them. I remember a rabbi in the States telling me that one of the ways of handling problems in a marriage was to ask for help from the other, so that when we finally leave this world we are better people because we have learnt something new. So instead of shouting when someone drops a bucket of water, all we need to say is "Where is the mop?" ➤

➤ This couple also agreed that one evening they would try and get the children to bed early, and, have a bath together. This would be their intimate time; neither of them wanted to rush into being sexual until they had resolved some of the resentments. Mary felt that it would help if they always tried holding hands when they were out walking. Within a month they regained their confidence and managed to prioritise their time together as a couple.

When we go to work, we sign a contract for a period of years; our work is continually assessed, giving us the opportunity to challenge new ways of thinking and adapting to different settings, people and circumstances. We would never keep the same contract for the whole of our working life. So why do it in relationships? I believe every six months we need to sit down with our partner and say "What is going well and what is not going well?" "What do we need to change?" "How can we help one another?"

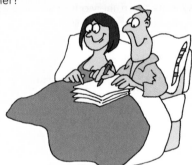

CASE STUDY 10

Liz and Simon had been married for 40 years when they turned up at the clinic together. Simon had recently undergone two knee replacements; since the surgery, he was worried about initiating sex. They had always had sex with Simon on top with his knees bent. Both of them had become worried that they might do some further damage to his knees if they continued to use these sexual positions. Liz was a quiet lady, who had never initiated sexual activity, and they had rarely spoken about sex throughout their marriage, even though it had occurred regularly. For the first time in their lives they had to try to find a sexual language, and both were embarrassed and anxious.

I explained how difficult it can be to change patterns of a lifetime and that finding a language to talk about sex can be difficult. I suggested they wrote down, individually, all the words they felt comfortable using to describe the vagina, penis, intercourse, etc and to choose a word that they were both comfortable using. They also purchased a video. This showed couples using different sexual positions. I asked them to do this exercise in the sitting room with their clothes on. They were to freeze the film once a position had been shown and try to copy it. I asked them to stay in the position for a few minutes and talk about whether they felt comfortable. They came back a few weeks later, full of ideas and with a changed repertoire.

CASE STUDY 11

Mary and Tom had been married for over 30 years, and had always enjoyed a good sex life. They came to the clinic anxious that their lovemaking had become very sporadic. This was of concern to them, especially as they were both fit and healthy and enjoyed intercourse.

They explained that their three children had recently moved back into the family home, to save money. Each of them now had a partner so the house was full, and the fridge always empty!

They felt embarrassed about having intercourse in case they were heard, even though they were aware that their children expected privacy and were sexually active. We made up a poster to place on their bedroom door. It said. "We are being intimate, please do not disturb". Six weeks later they returned, smiling!

Two of the children had moved out, and the other son had moved to the far end of the house. As soon as the sign was noticed, the children held a meeting and decided it was time for them to move on! Mary and Tom were delighted. There was food in the fridge, hot water in the tank, and they could watch whatever they wanted on TV!

They began to have more regular sexual activity again and agreed that it was important to talk to their children about intimacy issues. The sign on the door helped to initiate the discussion.

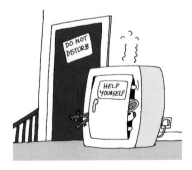

Many children feel that they should have access to their parents' bedroom at any time. As we get older, our children are horrified if we enter their room without knocking, but it is acceptable for them to have access to ours, often without knocking!

I am sure that, in years to come, many children will be living with their parents for longer. Therefore, we need to discuss intimacy issues directly with our children. It is very important that they grow up acknowledging the importance of a couple's time together, as this will be their relationship model for when they are older. So many young people presume that intimacy doesn't happen when bodies become old and wrinkly. We need to teach them that this is not so, otherwise many of us will be avoiding intimacy, and this will lead to resentments and loneliness.

Timing

Do you remember the days when you didn't look at your watch or worry what you should or ought to be doing? When you had that tremendous urge to be physically close and kiss and lie next to one another, perhaps leading to intercourse?

This relaxed attitude and easiness changes, and I very often hear couples saying "We just don't have any time for sex. We are so busy and so tired". It seems that sex has become a chore, hard work, difficult and unrewarding. Whenever I see a client with a sexual problem, I always ask them "when and what time do you normally initiate sex?"

So often these days it is late at night when too much food and alcohol has been consumed. Can you remember the last time you made love without having had a drink? Of course, alcohol can loosen your inhibitions and relax you, but it can also have a devastating effect on slowing down orgasm. Either it doesn't happen at all or it takes a long time to reach it. Women and men can complain of sore genitals, waking with a feeling of sexual frustration and a headache!

If you are experiencing sexual problems, I suggest you alter the timing of sex. It is very difficult to concentrate loving each others bodies when you are tired and anxious.

TOP TIPS

- Set the alarm and hour early, and use time to touch and caress one another
- Turn the television off early and go and have a bath together
- Go to bed in the afternoon
- Don't try and expect sex to be perfect late at night when you are tired and drunk

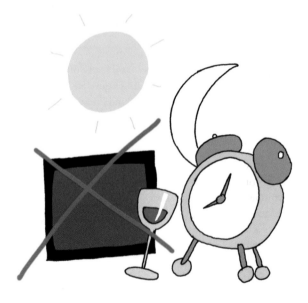

Ref: www.lovelifematters.co.uk

CHAPTER 10

Are we too old for sex?

VICTORIA

One of the frequent questions I get asked by men and women is "Do you think that we are too old to be having sex?" or "Is the cause of our erectile problems related to age?" The answer is simple. The ageing process does affect the sexual response, but the good news is that sexual activity can still occur as long as you remember that everything just takes a little longer. That means more foreplay, more creativity, more talking, which all leads to greater sensual pleasure. We need to stop focusing on genital arousal and think about stimulating one another in other ways, like mutual masturbation, massage, and enjoying one another's bodies without the need for vaginal penetration. I know that this can be difficult, because when we are young, getting sexually aroused just seems to happen, often without much stimulation. As we get older there is a need to change our sexual behaviour and have the courage to touch much more.

I don't believe that anyone is too old to be sexually intimate. Of course, a vagina can lose some of its elasticity and some women can experience a change in lubrication that can cause vaginal discomfort. A penis can also be affected with increasing age. It can lose some of its sensitivity. There is often a fall in testosterone levels, and there are vascular changes. Many men complain of a change in the orgasmic experience and less ejaculate. The old adage "If you don't use it, you lose it" is true for both men and women. The importance we attach to sex remains high even as we grow older. Around 80% of men and 60% of women between the ages of 40 and 80 still rate sex as an important part of their lives, and over half continue to have sex between one and six times per week.

Unfortunately, even though our interest to have sex remains strong, between the ages of 40 and 70 a man's risk of suffering ED increases threefold. So what happens when your partner's erection is not rigid enough for vaginal penetration and your arthritic knees means that you can't manage the same sexual positions as before? It is time to talk seriously to one another about how you manage sexual activity together. There is nothing to be anxious about. The chances are that you have been together for a very long time. You will only become wiser and more comfortable with one another after you have spoken about this important issue.

Some women feel that they have no need to have sex, but they do want a cuddle and to feel loved. Men still love to have that feeling of being able to gain an erection, even if it is a soft one and, yes, men can still orgasm with a soft penis. It makes men feel masculine to have some level of sexual response. The reality is that elderly men can have a sexual need but their penis doesn't always respond.

Whatever your age, it is still really important that you visit your doctor and tell him about your sexual difficulties. He can explain why your partner is having difficulty getting or even maintaining an erection. He can also advise about the advantage of using a vaginal lubricant. Although as a couple you may decide not to seek treatment, many couples are relieved to have talked about their anxieties with a health professional. There are so many excellent treatments available, from pills to vacuum pumps and even injection therapy. It is important to ensure that you have all the information and knowledge, before you decide to put sexual activity on the back burner.

Here are a few tips to remember to maintain sexual satisfaction with advancing age! Timing is important. Sex after a good night's sleep, or in the early afternoon is so much better than trying to stay awake after a long day when you are feeling tired. If it is in the morning, I suggest that you do get up and clean your teeth; kissing is so much more pleasant with a fresh mouth.

Sex is not a race. There is no need to hurry the event. Try not to be under performance pressure to orgasm quickly. Take it slowly and enjoy the sensuality of love making.

Be creative, and talk about different ways that you could please one another. If you are thinking of trying a different sexual position, first try it with your clothes on and see if you feel comfortable, then when you are naked with one another, you will feel less anxious.

If we don't discuss sexual activity when we are older, there is always the fear that a couple will lose the intimacy of the relationship. Everyone, whatever age they are, deserves to have a hug.

CASE STUDY 12

A man of 80 just wanted that loving feeling back. He had been sexually active with his wife for over 60 years and it was only in the last few months that the erections had not been satisfactory. Sexual closeness was a very valued commodity in their marriage, and their sadness caused them both to be tearful and anxious. Unfortunately, during the last six months both of them had experienced health problems and this contributed to their sexual difficulties.

I asked them to spend one afternoon a week caressing one another, and told them that they could experience that loving feeling and a rosy glow without an erection. Sometimes we have to adapt our sex lives in later life, but that loving feeling can still remain.

There is a story of a delightful man who had some erection problems. He thought that he would manage a lot better if his wife was a little more vocal in bed. His new wife was in her 70s, and wasn't too keen, but she agreed that for one night only she would encourage him by using some sexy words and sounds. That night she initiated sex, and said all the right things at the right time. At the next visit he said there had been no change to his erections. His wife with a smile on her face said, "I did exactly what he wanted, but he forgot to put his hearing aid in!" There was no second chance.

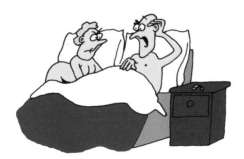

Staying intimate without sex

VICTORIA

When a man attends my clinic, I always ask him when he last had intercourse. For many, years have passed since they put their penis in their partner's vagina, or even attempted intercourse. I then ask when was the last time that you and your partner had a hug, kissed or cuddled. The majority of men tell me that hugs and kisses stopped about the same time that their ED problems started. The reason they give is that they feel it would be unfair to offer any kind of intimacy as they were unable to continue to engage in fulfilling sexual intercourse. When their partner has tried to be intimate in a non sexual way, they often respond by moving away, or going to sleep at a later time, or making some excuse that it is better for them to sleep separately. We are all incredibly clever at finding ways of avoiding sexual contact!

Of course, it is not always the men that avoid intimacy. Many women say that it is best to avoid any hugs because they don't want to embarrass their partners by reminding them that they are unable to have sexual intercourse. They tell their partners that their vagina is painful, or that their periods are very heavy, so that intercourse would be difficult, or they switch off their desire to have sex and make a conscious decision to live without intimacy rather than bring up a discussion about sex.

Is there such a thing as being intimate without sexual activity taking place? Intimacy is a word which women use more often than men. I think it describes those hugs and cuddles that are so important. Intimacy means being treasured, loved and cherished – it is that feeling we get when a man touches our arm or strokes our face for no other reason but to say that he really cares. Research has shown that some women prefer foreplay to vaginal penetration. Men need to know this, so that the focus of sex isn't just on the penis going inside the vagina. I think that men also love to have a hug or a cuddle, but some believe it is not manly to ask for a sensual touch without sex.

When men experience erection problems, they truly believe that it is not possible to be intimate without continuing to have sex. Therefore, if they are unable to gain an erection sufficient for intercourse to take place, they withdraw from intimate touch. I think that it is important that women explain to their partners that even though intercourse may not be possible, there are many other ways of showing someone that you love and cherish them. Sex is not all about penetration, although of course it is good to have a penis in a vagina; in fact, some men believe it is the only way for women to experience orgasm!

I believe that, sometimes, sexual problems can be used to our advantage. Whilst we wait for blood tests and treatment, we have the opportunity to reassess how we show our loved ones that we love them. Sometimes we get so used to intercourse that we forget there are other ways of being sexual.

Why not say to your partner "I know that it is difficult for us to have intercourse at the moment, but we can be sexual in other ways". Many men really enjoy pleasuring a woman to orgasm either with oral sex or by stimulating the clitoris with their hand. You could also have a bath together – there is real closeness involved when two naked bodies are touching one another.

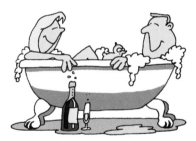

There are many vibrators on the market, so buying a clitoral stimulator can enhance the enjoyment. We all need a bit of variety in our lovemaking. Sometimes we need to be very clear about expressing ourselves about intimacy. I don't believe that any of us enjoys living without touch. It is one of the most important and valued ingredients of any relationship.

Ref: www.lovelifematters.co.uk

CHAPTER 11

Starting a new relationship after break up, divorce or death

VICTORIA

Any ending to a relationship can be traumatic and, of course, it varies as to why and how the ending occurred. One of the greatest problems is learning to have the confidence to try to trust again; after all, the pain of losing a partner can be so extreme that the thought of ever going through it again can bring such anxiety that it often feels better just to leave it alone.

What often happens is that we do engage in relationships, but we sabotage any future together by ensuring that the new partner has "something wrong" with them. It is like leaving the back door open, so that you can always escape. We don't allow ourselves any great depth of intimacy, so that we maintain the power in the relationship, and we end up going out with unobtainable partners, or people who have such a different set of values to ourselves that there would be no point in maintaining the relationship long term.

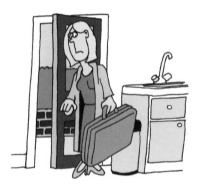

One of the common problems that my patients talk about is how are they going to restart their sex lives, especially if there has been a long gap between partners? There is an assumption that when we are older, or have had a previous long term relationship we should know what to do and when, without even checking anything out. What we don't realise is that, if we have been with one partner for many years, we get used to them. We know what to expect, how they touch, when they touch, what they like and what they don't. There is often an unspoken language about intimacy. We adapt our sex lives to fit in with our regular routines. When we are older, it all changes.

When we have the confidence to start a new relationship, we need to find a language to speak openly and clearly together. There is absolutely no point in making assumptions. Just because a partner was in a relationship for 30 years, it does not mean that he or she has ever had oral sex, or even touched the genitals. It can be terrifying for men or women to be asked to do some intimate act which they have never done before.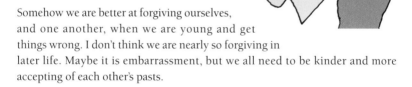

Somehow we are better at forgiving ourselves, and one another, when we are young and get things wrong. I don't think we are nearly so forgiving in later life. Maybe it is embarrassment, but we all need to be kinder and more accepting of each other's pasts.

I remember a man coming to see me and saying that his new partner wanted him to find the G spot, so she could have an orgasm. "What, and where, is it?" he asked. Another man told me that his new partner wanted him to maintain an erection for at least an hour: "How do I do that?" he asked.

Partners can be very demanding and, remember a man cannot fake sexual excitement and orgasm like women, so be kind and thoughtful.

CASE STUDY 13

Harry aged 60 attended the clinic; he had started a new relationship with a lady who had been widowed like himself. They had loss and grief in common, but he felt very uncomfortable when she started to kiss him, as he noticed that he wasn't getting an erection. She asked him what was wrong, and he said "Nothing", and, from sheer embarrassment, he had ended their friendship.

"What happens if she tells our friends at the club that I was not interested in her, or worse tells them that I couldn't get an erection. I don't think I can face anyone again."

This charming man had been widowed for 10 years, and had not had any sexual activity with a partner and had not masturbated at all during this time. When he had been with his wife they rarely spoke during sexual activity, erections had just happened and, to be honest, they were not very creative. He did not know whether his wife had enjoyed sex, but it had been fairly regular and had seemed pleasurable. This new lady was completely different; she was outspoken about her need for sex, and wanted him to touch and kiss her in daylight hours, and had even suggested using a vibrator! It was all just too much for Harry.

Harry also was on some tablets to help lower his blood pressure and he thought that his penis was getting smaller. He admitted that he was not comfortable using sexual words, or asking for intimacy.

I explained that it would be helpful to ask his doctor to examine him and check out that his penis was healthy. Harry had quite a large tummy and often men complain that their penis is getting smaller when in fact the fatty tissue round the tummy 'sucks up' some of the penis and, when they look in the mirror, it looks smaller. Low testosterone levels can also alter the size of the penis.

It is a good idea to have a blood pressure check and tell the doctor that you are thinking that you might be getting into an intimate relationship again. Your doctor can reassure you and advise you, so that you will feel more confident.

I told Harry that he was asking too much of himself to gain a perfect erection on just a first kiss, especially after being so sexually inactive. He agreed that if he had the courage to be intimate with anyone again, he would warn them about his "level of expertise". He agreed that, for the first few months, he would just cuddle, until both of them felt comfortable with one another. I told him that if women started to be demanding at the beginning of the relationship, it would set the scene for a long time to come. He had to decide whether he could cope with a partner's sexual demands, or not.

CHAPTER 12

Mending your sexual circuit

VICTORIA

Imagine going to work every day, using the same route; you know where all the traffic lights are, when there is likely to be a hold up, but you always reach your destination. Then imagine taking that route one day, and finding that the road is closed. You have to look at a map to find another way to reach your destination. It takes time, you try another route and yet again you are stopped by road works. Time passes, you get agitated, cross, desperate to find a way through, and then you just give up and go home.

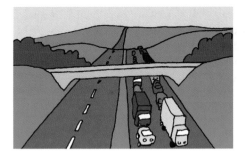

This is what it can be like for a man experiencing a sexual problem. For many years he takes for granted being able to get a good erection so that he can be intimate with a loved one. He knows what to do, what will happen, and the outcome. Then one day, the penis does not respond, or if it does, it doesn't stay up for very long or the ejaculation comes much quicker than he would like.

All hell lets loose. He may panic. Women can fake an orgasm, but men who want to have penetrative sex need a rigid erection.

Partners are only too well aware when a man's sexual response goes wrong or changes. It seems that if we start being intimate and think it will go wrong, the message is transferred into our male partner's brain. He senses our concern, and once again the erection subsides.

It is so worthwhile talking to your doctor. When the sexual circuit becomes confused it no longer works efficiently. It is like a circuit that has a loose wire. Treatments are now available which will help to overcome the symptoms.

Sex is at its best when the brain, the genitals and the whole of the body, responds with pleasure; when the genitals do not respond, the brain panics. It only takes one second for the brain to acknowledge that something is wrong, for the genitals to stop responding. It is like one sexual circuit working within your brain, and another in your genitals. We are now able to use treatments to help the genitals respond. Of course, they need stimulation, but the positive response reinforces a positive feeling in the brain and the two circuits often link up again.

There have been cases of using a low dose of an ED treatment to challenge the arousal response to respond differently. It is so easy to get demoralised or embarrassed and just give up, like the travel analogy. I make a plea to all those men out there: DO NOT GIVE UP. There are specialists who will empathise, and treatments that will help. There is no need to turn back.

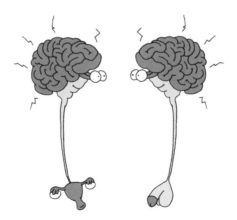

CHAPTER 13

The internet and those worries

VICTORIA

Here is a typical story:

"I was in the garden the other day, and my husband said he was busy on the computer. When I went upstairs I found him accessing a site of naked women, which completely shocked me. He quickly switched it off, but I am sure that he has been on the site before, even though he assures me that he hasn't. What am I to do?"

These terrible fears escalate into worries like "What if the children are looking on the computer and see in the history that a sex site has been accessed?" "Is my partner meeting or in contact with any of the people on the site?" "Is he going to want me to do certain sexual acts which he is watching on screen?" "What other sexual secrets does he have?"

There are many websites which show erotic material / pornography and even if you don't want to believe it many men, and women, now access these sites. Partly, it is probably because it is easier than going out to buy a magazine or DVD. After all, you have to be quite tall to pick up a magazine from the top shelf these days!

When a man experiences an erection problem, he often tries to arouse himself alone using some erotica. It is a way of checking out whether the penis is working. We all have our views about sexual activity, what we will and won't ever do sexually, and what we think is appropriate, and I don't want to tell you what you should think or do, but …

If you have noticed that your partner is accessing some pornography and you are uncomfortable about it, talk to him. Explain your discomfort and worries, and negotiate some sort of compromise. Please do go and find a therapist to talk to.

If you don't, your worries can easily spiral and become overwhelming, and you can end up worrying unnecessarily.

If you are using websites to access information on sexual issues, I suggest you use the resources file at the end of this book. Never buy anything from a website unless you are sure that your information is not going to be sold to another company without your knowledge or consent. Receiving literature from a variety of other companies can be embarrassing.

Remember too, that many of the drugs sold over the internet may be counterfeit. You must have a health check up before you start using any drugs, especially when they are for erection problems. Always tell your doctor if you are taking any medication which he has not prescribed, as it could interact with other drugs.

There are problems about arousing oneself always using erotica; it can get to be a habit and the vigorous stimulation with both hands is certainly very different from a soft wet vagina. The brain can get slightly confused and so adjusting to a real body can cause complications.

Some men can feel threatened and lose their confidence when watching pornography. Their expectations of how they ought to be cause an enormous amount of performance anxiety. They see a very large penis on screen and lots of ejaculate coming again and again. They think that their partners will love them more if their penis was bigger, and if they could maintain an erection and ejaculate for hours on end. It is important to have sexual expectations but they must be realistic.

I have said before that the more variety we have in your sex lives, the greater the chance of maintaining sexual intimacy into our old age. So watching a sexy video together can be fun as long as you have agreed about the content beforehand.

CHAPTER 14

Visiting your GP or a sex therapist: what to expect

MIKE

What to expect when visiting your GP

A doctor will try to obtain as much diagnostic information about the sexual problem as possible, including your specific concerns and symptoms. They will want to know what interventions have been tried to date, and the results of these interventions. They will enquire about your current medical problems and medications and about all past relevant medical and surgical treatments. Clearly, the doctor may wish to explore important psychological issues and relevant information about your relationship and any health problems with your partner.

You may be given a Sexual Health Inventory for Men (SHIM) which is a questionnaire to fill in (see appendix II). All patients with ED should undergo a full medical assessment, particularly focusing on risk factors such as cigarette smoking, high blood pressure, alcohol intake, drug abuse and hormone problems such as low levels of thyroid hormone or testosterone. Laboratory tests are usually kept to a minimum but will include blood glucose, lipid profile and morning serum testosterone.

The doctor will almost certainly encourage you to come with your partner if possible. The issue of embarrassment is very important in sexual health care. It deters men and women from seeking treatment and adopting healthy behaviour and it deters staff from broaching topics such as sexuality. There are many reasons for doctors and nurses not taking the initiative in discussing sexual problems. Most doctors and nurses are familiar with basic history taking, but are uncertain about how to obtain information on a patient's sexual function in a non-threatening way. Other factors include a lack of time, and incorrect perceptions about age, gender and culture of the patient. There is often a belief that the patient will initiate discussions if they are worried about a problem.

Surveys have shown the patients actually want, and expect, to be asked about their sexual problems, and many patients who find it difficult to initiate the discussion themselves are in fact desperate to be asked, and thus be saved the embarrassment of raising the subject themselves.

VICTORIA

What to expect when you visit a sex therapist

I sometimes imagine what it would be like to visit me, a sex and relationship therapist working within an NHS clinic. If I was a man experiencing sexual problems would I ever have the courage to follow a woman who is a complete stranger down a corridor into a small consulting room and discuss the intimate side of my sex life? The answer is probably "No"! I have the utmost respect for all those men who have followed me; I have never lost anyone on the way, although I always look behind me, perhaps someone will one day think to themselves "This is all just too much". I admire my patients' courage, and value them immensely.

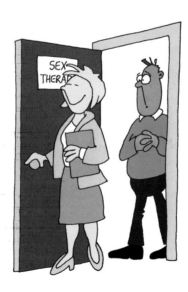

Once we sit down, I tell my patients that there will be no genital examination with me. I am fortunate that all my patients have been examined by a GP before they attend the clinic. There is always a sense of relief that at least they can keep their clothes on throughout my consultation. I explain that I am a qualified sex therapist who deals specifically with sexual problems and, in particular, erection problems. I think they find it comforting to know that their symptoms will be taken seriously. I ask them if they will tell me their story. All my patients have completed a questionnaire prior to the appointment, and this helps to focus the session on their specific difficulty. That way, I can also make sure that I have all the appropriate support leaflets available.

Once I have listened to all the symptoms, I will ask what they think is the cause and what they think will make it better. Many men believe their erection problems are related to recent ill health, medication, surgery or loss of a partner. Some feel that it may be age, or that they have been out of a relationship for such a long time, that their erections will never work again.

I organise blood tests, usually cholesterol and blood sugar, as well as doing investigations such as blood pressure and urine analysis. We talk about lifestyle, partners, and discuss the most appropriate treatment.

Some men have been suffering a very long time and, if there are no contraindications and they have no objections, and the partner is in agreement, we will discuss the possible use of an oral treatment. When they return four weeks later, we review the blood test results and the outcome of the treatment. All my patients' partners are invited to attend the appointments. Certainly the outcome of the treatment is better if they are seen as a couple.

Loss of sexual activity leads to immense distress and intense sadness. Many have lived without a hug or cuddle for years because they cannot sustain an erection. A consultation is so worthwhile; it is an opportunity to talk about sex in a safe and confidential environment and, most of all, to discover that there is always a way forward. Of course, other sex therapists work in different ways, but the outcome is generally the same.

All you need to remember is that there is no need to panic, and I can promise you that the consultation will be worthwhile.

CASE STUDY 14

"I get on really well with my new partner; we have been together six months now. Both of us have had previous marriages, and other relationships, so I guess we both feel quite sexually experienced. Well, the first few times we had sex, it was OK. I think all that lust added to the excitement. Now we see each other more regularly and, over the past few months, whenever we have had sex, his erection 'goes down' just after penetration, but sometimes he can't even stuff it in! I feel embarrassed and, to be honest, he is devastated.

At our age, life is too short to hang around waiting for things to change. So, we contacted our doctor and he performed some blood tests, then said he would refer us to a sex therapist. We were sent a questionnaire, which really helped us both to focus on what the problem was, and it even asked about how I felt! After all – it takes two to tango! I thought that it was entirely my fault; after all, I'm getting older. The questionnaire helped us to talk about this, and we felt a lot closer.

Both of us sat anxiously in the waiting room, wondering if everyone knew that we were there because we weren't having sex! Actually, it was OK. The lady called our names and introduced herself. She listened to the story, and thanked us for completing the questionnaire. She also checked all the blood test results.

It was so good to talk to someone, confidentially, about how we had both reacted to the erection problems. We had both been rejected by partners in the past, so this problem brought back some of those memories.

We had some counselling and medication. My partner was found to have high cholesterol, and erection problems are sometimes the first symptom of this. The erections are fine now. We feel so pleased with ourselves for acting quickly. Life's too short to live without a cuddle, and when men don't have erections they often back off from intimacy. We both deserved the best, and now we have it."

CASE STUDY 15

"When I met my partner we had regular sex. It seemed OK at the time; after all, that's what happens when you first start a relationship. Then it just seemed to me that he wanted sex all the time. I felt tired and irritated that we couldn't just go to sleep and cuddle. I used to say, "Why can't we just have a cuddle and no sex." He would then turn over and we wouldn't talk for few days. I found these days unbearable and I felt angry and resentful.

Sometimes I used to give in and have sex and then I decided that I would just say "No".

We started going to bed at different times. It was almost like living as brother and sister.

One day, I was reading an article about women not feeling like sex and it suggested that you talked your GP or contacted a counsellor. I felt too embarrassed to talk to my doctor so I looked on the internet and found an experienced counsellor who specialised in relationship and sex problems.

My husband wasn't too keen about going to the first appointment. "Why do we need to talk about this with someone else, when all you have to do is to have sex more regularly?" You can imagine my reply!

In the end I said I would go on my own as I couldn't put up with his moods any more. On the day of the appointment, I was so anxious. I didn't know what to wear, and all my thoughts were muddled. Surely a sex therapist would be having sex all the time, and would think I was just being difficult.

In fact, the moment I met her I felt really comfortable. She smiled and showed me to the room. She introduced herself and we agreed that my session would remain confidential. She asked me to tell her the whole story. I felt heard for the very first time. It was so good to explain what it was like not wanting sex. I realised I was quite frightened that my marriage was at risk. She made no judgements at all and I felt I could just be me.

She thought it would be a good idea if my husband was also initially seen alone. Then we could both decide whether to come back for some couple therapy. I spoke to my husband and I couldn't believe that he agreed to go on his own.

We have now had four sessions together. We are much happier as a couple and I feel sure that we will find a way of handling our different needs for sex. At least we can have a cuddle now."

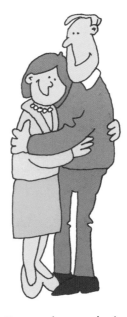

Everyone deserves a hug!

Ref: www.lovelifematters.co.uk

Appendix I

Useful contacts

British Association of Sexual and Relationship Therapy
Tel: 0208 543 2707
Email: info@basrt.org.uk
www.basrt.org,.uk

Sexual Dysfunction Association
Helpline: 0870 7743571
www.sda.uk.net/

Relate
0845 130 4010
www.relate.org.uk

Vibrators / sex toys
www.traceycoxshop.com

Diabetes UK
Care Line – 0207 424 1030

British Heart Foundation
0870 6006566

InContact
(for help with bladder problems)
Tel : 0870 770 3246
Email: info@incontact.org
www.incontact.org

Other useful websites:

www.erection.advice.co.uk
www.informED.org.uk
www.sortedin10.co.uk

Manufacturers' websites:
For more information about ED in general and the specific treatments go to:

Viagra:
www.viagra.com/
Cialis:
www.cialis.com/common_pages/fastfacts.jsp
Levitra:
www.levitra.com/about.html

Appendix II

The Sexual Health Inventory for Men (SHIM)
From http://www.ucof.com/files/SHIM.pdf)

Patient Name: .... **Today's Date:** ....

Patient Instructions
Sexual health is an important part of an individual's overall physical and emotional well-being. Erectile dysfunction, also known as impotence, is one type of very common medical condition affecting sexual health. Fortunately, there are many different treatment options for erectile dysfunction. This questionnaire is designed to help you and your doctor identify if you may be experiencing erectile dysfunction. If you are, you may choose to discuss treatment options with your doctor.

Each question has several possible responses. Circle the number of the response that **best describes** your own situation. Please be sure that you select one and only one response for **each question**.

1. How do you rate your confidence that you could get and keep an erection?

Very low	Low	Moderate	High	Very high
1	2	3	4	5

2. When you had erections with sexual stimulation, how often were your erections hard enough for penetration (entering your partner)?

No sexual activity	Almost never/never	A few times (much less than half the time)	Sometimes (about half the time)	Most times (much more than half the time)	Almost always/always
0	1	2	3	4	5

3. During sexual intercourse, how often were you able to maintain your erection after you had penetrated (entered) your partner?

Did not attempt intercourse	Almost never/never	A few times (much less than half the time)	Sometimes (about half the time)	Most times (much more than half the time)	Almost always/always
0	1	2	3	4	5

4. During sexual intercourse, how difficult was it to maintain your erection to completion of intercourse?

Did not attempt intercourse	Extremely difficult	Very difficult	Difficult	Slightly difficult	Not difficult
0	1	2	3	4	5

5. When you attempted sexual intercourse, how often was it satisfactory for you?

Did not attempt intercourse	Almost never/never	A few times (much less than half the time)	Sometimes (about half the time)	Most times (much more than half the time)	Almost always/always
0	1	2	3	4	5

Add the numbers corresponding to questions 1-5. TOTAL: ....

The Sexual Health Inventory for Men further classifies ED severity with the following breakpoints: 1–7 Severe ED; 8-11 Moderate ED; 12–16 Mild to Moderate ED; 17–21 Mild ED.

References

1. Kirby RS, Holmes S, Carson C. Male Erectile Dysfunction. Oxford: Health Press, 1997.
2. British Heart Foundation Statistic Database, 2002.
3. Wilson PK, Farday PS, Froelicher V, eds. Cardiac rehabilitation: Adult Fitness and Exercise Testing. Philadelphia: Lea & Fabiger, 1981.
4. Adapted from information provided by the Prostate Research Campaign UK: www.prostate-research.org.uk
5. Music for Two (referred to throughout): www.lovelifematters.co.uk
6. The section on sex and the heart is based on the two Princeton Consensus papers, and many of our observations are drawn from discussions we have had with, and the written work of, other experts in sexual medicine, whose opinions we value and appreciate.

Appendix III

Pelvic Floor Exercises for Women

- How to do your Pelvic Floor Muscle Exercises
- Vaginal Cones
- Biofeedback
- Electrical Stimulation

How to do your Pelvic Floor Muscle Exercises

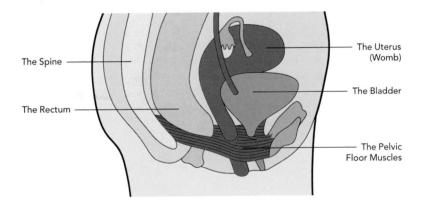

The Spine

The Rectum

The Uterus (Womb)

The Bladder

The Pelvic Floor Muscles

The pelvic floor is a large sling (or hammock) of muscles and other tissues stretching across the floor of the pelvis. It is attached to your pelvic side walls, your pubic bone in front, and to the coccyx (the tail end of the spine) behind. It forms your "undercarriage". The openings from your bladder (urethra), your bowels (rectum) and your womb (vagina) all pass through your pelvic floor.

What does it do?

- It supports your pelvic organs and abdominal contents, especially when you are standing or exerting yourself.
- It supports the bladder to help it stay closed. It actively squeezes when you cough or sneeze to help avoid leaking. When the muscles are not working effectively you may suffer from leaking ("urinary incontinence"), and/or urgent or frequent need to pass urine.
- It is used to control wind and when "holding on" with your bowels.
- It has an important sexual function, helping to increase sexual satisfaction both for yourself and your partner during sexual intercourse.

How to do pelvic floor muscle exercises

Exercise 1

Tighten the muscles around your back passage, vagina and front passage and lift up and squeeze inside as if trying to stop passing wind and urine at the same time. You need to concentrate on using the correct muscles, so don't squeeze your legs together or tighten your buttocks. However, many people find they tighten their lower stomach muscles at the same time, so if you hollow your lower stomach at the same time, that is OK -- the muscles are helping one another.

It is most important not to hold your breath: just breathe normally.

Have a go! How many seconds can you 'lift and squeeze" the pelvic floor muscles for? Try holding them as long and as strong as you can. Rest for 4 seconds and then repeat the contraction as many times as you can up to a maximum of 10 contractions. Gradually increase the time that you can hold each contraction, aiming for 10 second holds.

Try doing these exercises in a slow and controlled way with a rest of 4 seconds between each muscle contraction. Practise your maximum number of held contractions (up to 10) about three or four times each day.

Exercise 2

It is important to be able to work these muscles quickly to help them react to sudden stresses from coughing, laughing or exercise that put pressure on the bladder. So you need to practise some quick contractions, drawing in the pelvic floor and holding for just one second before releasing the muscles. Do these in a steady manner: aim for a strong muscle tightening with each contraction up to a maximum of 10 times.

Aim to do one set of slow contractions (exercise 1) followed by one set of quick contractions (exercise 2) three or four times each day.

Get into the habit!

Get into the habit of doing the exercises. Link doing them to some everyday activities - for example, do them after emptying your bladder or whenever you turn on a tap. Or keep a simple exercise diary (you could have an unlabelled simple tick chart on a kitchen pin board) to help you remember. Practise the exercises when you are lying, sitting and especially standing. In is also important to get into the habit of tightening your pelvic floor muscles before and during activities that are likely to make you leak - such as getting up from a chair, coughing, sneezing or lifting.

How long should I do them for?

Pelvic floor muscle exercises should give optimum results with regular exercise within 3 to 6 months, but you should continue them at least once a day for life to safeguard against problems recurring.

You are strongly recommended to seek help from a health professional if you see little or no change in your symptoms after trying these exercises on your own for three months.

If you find it difficult to exercise your pelvic floor muscles by your self...

...you could consider the following techniques.

Vaginal Cones

These are small weights which can be used by women to help with their pelvic floor exercises. The idea is to place an appropriate weight cone in the vagina and use the pelvic floor muscles to hold it there. By using it for 15-20 minutes at a time while walking around at home you will give your pelvic floor muscles some good exercise.

Some makes come as a set of cones of different weights, others as a single cone that unscrews to allow you to put in different weights. In either case you start by using the weight of cone that you can keep in for a short period once or twice a day, gradually increasing the weight, frequency and length of time you use them. (Full instructions are supplied with them.) You can buy cones directly from the manufacturers or from some branches of Boots the Chemist: see our Products Directory for information. They cost from £20 upwards.

Vaginal weighted cones can be ineffective if they are not in the right position. They will not work if you have anything more than a minor degree of prolapse. Some women find that the cone either slips out of the vagina almost immediately no matter how good the pelvic floor muscles are or else stays lodged in the vagina with no muscle work required to keep it in place. In fact, the evidence seems to suggest that using cones does not add any benefit if you are doing your pelvic floor muscle exercises properly - but they may help you to do the exercises correctly and many women say they have been useful.

Overall it is recommended that you talk to your nurse or physiotherapist before you try to use weighted cones.

The nurse/physiotherapist can instruct you in their proper use - and make sure you are doing your exercises right. Phone the Continence Foundation Helpline for a start.

Biofeedback

Biofeedback techniques includes anything that increases knowledge of your own body by sight, touch, sound etc. It can help as a motivator, give incentive and make pelvic floor muscle exrcises more interesting. This is usually used along with pelvic floor exercises for symptoms of stress incontinence and/or overactive bladder.

- A mirror can be used to see if there is any inwards movement of the perineum (the area between the vagina and back passage) when you contract your pelvic floor muscles. If you see any bulging, stop and seek further help from a specialist nurse/physiotherapist as you may be doing something that could cause problems.

- A sexual partner can give feedback.

- Vaginal cones may be used as described above.

- The use of more sophisticated machinery using pressure and other types of equipment. This is usually used as an adjunct to pelvic floor exercises for symptoms of stress and/or urge incontinence to show how your pelvic floor muscles are working - and hopefully improving. The most sophisticated type of biofeedback needs to be used under the supervision of a specialised practitioner, usually a specialist physiotherapist or specialist nurse. It is not directly beneficial in itself - but it does help you (if you need help) to do your pelvic floor exercises properly.

Pelvic Floor Exercises for Men

How to do your Pelvic Floor Muscle Exercises

Men experience a variety of problems with their urinary system, leading to unwanted leakage of urine. Some also have difficulty controlling wind or leakage from the bowels. Often this is due to a weakness of the muscles of the pelvic floor, which have an important function in preventing these troublesome conditions. In particular, pelvic floor exercises have been shown to be effective following surgery on the prostate and when men experience a dribble after passing water.

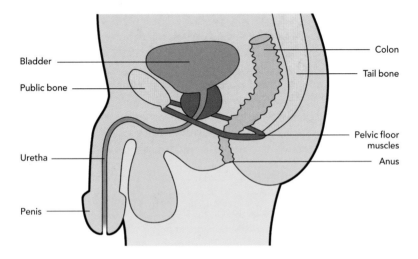

The floor of the pelvis is made up of layers of muscle and other tissues stretching from like a hammock across the floor of the pelvis and attached to your tail bone (coccyx) at the back and to the pubic bone in front. The urethra (bladder outlet) and the rectum (back passage) pass through the pelvic floor muscles. The hammock of muscles and other tissues supports the bladder and the bowel and plays an important role in bladder and bowel control.

Why the Pelvic Floor Muscles get Weak

The pelvic floor muscles can be weakened by:
- some operations for an enlarged prostate gland
- continual straining to empty your bowels, usually due to constipation
- a chronic cough, such as smoker's cough or chronic bronchitis or asthma
- being overweight.

Although there is no research evidence, it is thought by many that lack of general fitness and persistent heavy lifting tend to result in weakening of the pelvic floor.

Neurological damage (e.g., after a stroke or spinal injury, or resulting from multiple sclerosis or other conditions) can also produce poor pelvic muscle function. People in this group need to seek advice from a healthcare professional.

Pelvic Floor Muscle Exercises

You can improve control of your bladder and bowel by doing exercises to strengthen your pelvic floor muscles. These exercises may also be useful in conjunction with a bladder retraining programme aimed at improving bladder control in people who experience the urgent need to pass urine frequently and may not always "make it in time".

How to Identify your Pelvic Floor Muscles

The first thing to do is to identify correctly the muscles that need to be exercised.
1. Sit or lie comfortably with muscles of your thighs, buttocks and abdomen relaxed.
2. Tighten the ring of muscle around the back passage as if you are trying to control diarrhoea or wind. Relax it. Practise this movement several times until you are sure you are exercising the correct muscle. Do not hold your breath: keep breathing normally. You need to concentrate on using the correct muscles. Do not tighten your buttocks or thighs. Some people find they pull in the lower stomach muscles as well and this is OK because the muscles are helping one another.

3. In order to contract your pelvic floor muscles it may help to imagine you are passing urine and trying to stop the flow mid-stream, then restarting it. If your technique is correct, each time that you tighten your pelvic floor muscles you may feel the base of your penis move up slightly towards your abdomen.

4. If you are unable to feel a definite squeeze and lift action of your pelvic floor muscles, you should seek professional help to get your pelvic floor muscles working correctly. Even men with very weak pelvic floor muscles can be taught these exercises by a physiotherapist or continence advisor with expertise in this area. See "Seeking Help" below.

Doing Your Pelvic Floor Muscle Exercises

Now that you can feel the muscles working, you can start to exercise them:

1. Tighten and draw in strongly the muscles around the anus and the urethra all at once. Lift them up inside. Try and hold this contraction strongly as you count to five, then release slowly and relax for a few seconds. You should have a definite feeling of "letting go".

2. Repeat ("squeeze and lift") and relax. It is important to rest in between each contraction. If you find it easy to hold the contraction for a count of five, try to hold for longer - up to ten seconds.

3. Repeat this as many times as you are able up to a maximum of 8-10 squeezes. Make each tightening a strong, slow and controlled contraction.

4. Now do five to ten short, fast, but strong contractions, pulling up and immediately letting go.

5. Do this whole exercise routine at least 3-4 times every day. You can do it in a variety of positions - lying, sitting, standing, walking.

6. While doing the exercises:
   - DO NOT hold your breath.
   - DO NOT push down instead of squeezing and lifting up.

Do your exercises carefully. The quality is important. Fewer good exercises will be more beneficial than many half-hearted ones.

Make the Exercises a Daily Routine

Once you have learnt how to do these exercises, they should be done regularly, giving each set your full attention. It might be helpful to have regular times during the day for doing the exercises - for example, after going to the toilet, when having a drink, when lying in bed. You will wish to tighten your pelvic floor muscles also while you are getting up from a chair, coughing or lifting. Some men find that by tightening before they undertake such activities they assist themselves in regaining control.

Good results take time. In order to build up your pelvic floor muscles to their maximum strength you will need to work hard at these exercises. You will probably not notice an improvement for several weeks and you will not reach your maximum performance for a few months.

When you have recovered control of your bladder or bowel you should continue doing the at least once a day for life.

Other Tips to Help Your Pelvic Floor

- Avoid constipation and prevent any straining during a bowel movement.
- Seek medical advice for hay-fever, asthma or bronchitis to reduce sneezing and coughing.
- Keep your weight within the right range for your height and age.
- Share the lifting of heavy loads.

Seeking Help

To achieve your best results or if your problems persist despite doing the exercises, you may need to seek help professional help from your GP, a physiotherapist or a specialist continence nurse - you can obtain details of your local NHS specialist continence service from the InContact website www.incontact.org. You may be advised to use some additional technique, such as biofeedback or electrical stimulation.

Biofeedback

This is usually used along with pelvic floor muscle exercises for symptoms of stress and/or urge incontinence, although there has been no clear research to prove its effectiveness in men. It requires the use of mechanical or electronic equipment to provide you with visual feedback about how your muscles are working - and hopefully improving. Biofeedback needs to be used in conjunction with a specialised practitioner, usually a specialist physiotherapist or specialist nurse.

These exercises are reproduced with kind permission of the Continence Foundation:

www.incontact.org

Index